Written From The Heart

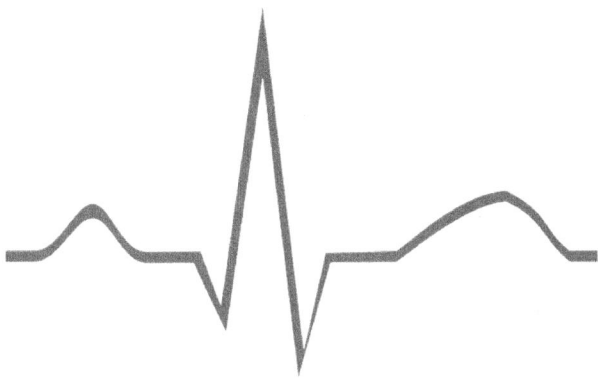

My Journey From Hospital to Healing with Practical Advice

Joanna Montagna Torreano

Copyright © 2020, Joanna Montagna Torreano.

All names and places are fictitious. Any similarity to people or places is coincidental. The fictitious names of the doctors represent their practice specialties.

Photo of the Spirometer provided by the author.

Cover image of EKG pattern from clker.com.

Book design by Mike Miller, pubyourbook@gmail.com.

ISBN: 9798644576500

Dedication

To my husband, Paul, who firmly and gently pointed me in all the right directions. To all the medical staff, without you, I wouldn't be here.

Table of Contents

Primary Beginning	1
Dr. Heart Appointment	5
Echocardiogram	9
1st Echo Results	13
Echo Testing – Six Months Later	15
2nd Echo Test	17
Dr. Heart 2nd Echo Results	19
Dr. Surgeon Initial Call	22
Dr. Surgeon Visit	25
Dr. Surgeon Consultation	29
Angiogram Appointment	33
Waiting on an Angiogram	35
Before Angiogram	37
Before Angiogram - Part 2	42
During Angiogram	46
After the Angiogram	49
Phone Call to Dr. Surgeon	51
Admission - Part 1	53
Admission - Part 2	56
Hospital Procedures	59
Holding	62
Roll-'Er-In	65
ICU - Part 1	67
ICU - Part 2	69
Doctor Visit	71
Helplessness	73
Regular Room	75
Visitors	82
From Nun to Married	84
The Spirometer	88

Consequences	90
Leaving the Hospital	91
Visiting Nurse Appointment	96
VNA Visit - Amy	99
Pre-Cardiac Rehab	105
Sometimes Family is Right	107
Embarrassed	110
Cardiac Rehab	112
Cardiac Flunkie	115
High Blood Pressure	117
Dr. Heart - High Blood Pressure	120
Return to Cardiac Rehab	123
Last Day of Cardio Rehab	126
Post-Stress Test	129
Cardio without Monitoring	132
Eye Appointment for Black Dot	134
Linda	138
May 25, 2019 - Check-up Echo	141
Echo Result May 2019	144
June 6, 2019	147
March 31, 2020 – A Sense of Urgency	150
Glossary	157
About The Author	158
Book Club Discussion Topics	159

Primary Beginning

After the annual exam, Dr. Primary closed her laptop, shook my hand, and looked at me eye to eye. "Don't worry Joanna, I'm just being careful."

She was more than careful, she was right. I had a problem.

My 2 o'clock appointment was pretty much on time. Lynn, the nurse, greeted me. I heard the squeak of the door as the nurse walked into the waiting room. "Joanna?" she said.

I packed up my book and headed her way. Once we reached the scale, I stepped on and watched her move the weight to the right, until it balanced my weight. Not bad, I said to myself. I was within normal ranges.

"Room 2," she said pointing. I entered and she patted the examining table, "Can you hop up?"

"With effort."

"How have you been?" Lynn questioned.

"Good, real good," I replied with a conviction that I shouldn't have had.

"Any changes in medication?" she asked, as she began to enter data on her computer.

"No, I don't take anything."

Placing the blood pressure cuff on my left arm, she pumped the bulb to add air. As the valve released, it sounded like a balloon wanting a little more time at life. Then the pulse oximeter on my finger indicated my oxygen saturation and heart rate.

"Everything is normal," she said.

But that was meaningless to me since I didn't know what normal was anyway.

Before going on to the next patient, Lynn said, "Dr. Primary will be with you shortly. Do you have any questions for her?"

"No, I'm good."

She opened the door, turned, and said, "It's good to see you again, Joanna."

"You too, Lynn."

I hopped off the table, grabbed my book, and tried to read it, but I couldn't focus. Instead, I looked at the photos on the wall and read the announcements that were posted.

I could hear someone in the next room, yet I couldn't catch the conversation, which made me feel good that mine wouldn't be shared either. I heard the door next to me open and close. Footsteps followed with the sound of a stool scraping on the floor. Dr. Primary was probably taking notes.

Having a good book and being able to read the book are two different events. There is something intimidating about being vulnerable and checked over even though I knew this was just routine.

A slight knock on the door and Dr. Primary walked in. "Hi, Joanna," she said extending her right hand to shake mine. "Lynn said everything looked normal. What questions do you have for me?" she asked as she put her computer down and looked at me.

"Nothing, I'm just here for my annual check-up."

"Okay, let's get started."

She opened up her computer to a screen where I saw my photo and she began asking me routine questions. There was nothing out of the ordinary and she slowly got off her stool and began a physical exam.

Eyes, ears, nose, and checking for any swelling of the feet or hands. Everything was normal. Next, the stethoscope. She placed the listening tubes in her ears and gently placed the disc-shaped object on my heart. As if on cue, my heart's thump seemed to get louder as if wanting to be recognized.

"Can you take a deep breath and hold it please?" she asked.

I complied. She adjusted the stethoscope as if she needed to hear it correctly. "Take another deep breath." Although she tried to keep her expression normal, I felt that something was wrong. Her left eye squinted upward and she cocked her head to the right.

"Everything seems fine. I'd like you to make an appointment with a cardiologist just to make sure. Nothing to be alarmed about, but your mitral valve needs to be heard by a competent cardiologist."

I immediately went into overdrive, "Why? What did you hear?"

"Oh, it's probably nothing, just a good idea to get it checked out."

She sat down and typed a few notes on the computer. Looking up, she asked, "Do you have a specific doctor you'd like to go to or would you like a recommendation?" she asked.

Taking a deep breath and quickly letting it out, I said, "Give me a name of someone you'd go to."

She smiled and handed me a sheet of paper where she had written, Dr. Heart. "He's the best. If I had a question, I'd go to him." She paused, "Would you like us to make an appointment or would you prefer to make it on your own?"

Her accommodating suggestion, which would normally bring comfort, brought distress. My mind was overly engaged. The calendar I kept was at home hanging on the wall. Being recently retired, I had no 9-to-5 job I had to report to, but I needed time to process this information.

"How about I make it and if I have a problem, I'll let you know?" I asked.

"Sounds good," she replied.

She closed the laptop, shook my hand. Before walking away, she looked at me and waited to make eye contact before saying, "Don't worry Joanna, I just like to be thorough."

Her attention to detail saved me from a life with an oxygen tank.

My Lesson Learned

Keep your yearly check-up appointment. You may feel fine but it's like wearing glasses. Once you put them on, you realize how clearly you can see. Same with a check-up, you may feel fine, but things could be off.

Dr. Heart Appointment

Hesitantly I picked up the phone and dialed 555-5555. It rang a few times before I heard, "Doctors' offices, can you hold?"

"Yes." *Here we go* I muttered to myself.

The music came on immediately. I placed my phone on speaker so I could continue munching on my breakfast. Surprised at the promptness, I heard, "Thank you for holding. My name is Renee. How may I help you?"

Swallowing my last morsel of cereal, I responded, "I was asked by my medical doctor, Dr. Primary, to make an appointment with Dr. Heart."

"May I ask what this is for?" Renee asked.

"She didn't like the sound of my mitral valve." I hated saying it because it made it more real.

I could hear the busyness of the office through the phone. Voices in the background and ringing phones came through my line. "Boy, my computer is slow today. Sorry about that," she said.

"No problem." I took that opportunity to swallow more tea.

I pictured the computer mouse and keyboard activity. "Well, it looks like Dr. Heart had a cancellation for next Wednesday at 2 o'clock. Does that work?"

"Sure," I replied. I took another long sip of hot tea and felt the warmness going down.

"Let me ask you a few questions to get you started on paperwork."

She proceeded to ask about my medical insurance and any medications I was taking. We finished up quickly.

Before hanging up, she said, "Please get here 15 minutes before your appointment to complete your paperwork."

"Oh, I forgot to ask, do I need a referral?" I questioned.

A few clicks on her computer and her response came quickly, "No, not with your insurance. Do you know where we are located?"

"No," I answered.

As she provided the details I felt two emotions, calm and nervous. My mind skipped around like a child chasing a butterfly.

Before hanging up, she said, "We look forward to seeing you next Wednesday at 2 o'clock."

Getting up from the chair, I put the information on my wall calendar. No computer reminder, just an old-fashioned wall hanging calendar. I took a deep sigh and continued on with my day with mixed emotions. Questions that popped into my mind; I pushed them down like a hammer on a nail.

Who is this guy? Why was I able to get in so quickly? Did I trust my primary enough to go with her recommendation? For that, I could say yes. But the other questions haunted me for a week.

My husband, who hates going to doctor's offices more than I do, wanted to come with me. He's a pharmacist and asks questions I don't even think of. His tapping foot while staying in the waiting room I learned to tolerate. *Isn't that what you do in a marriage?* I reminded myself that he chose to come with me as he bounced his leg up and down. True to the receptionist's words, there was more paperwork to fill out. Some of the questions had already been answered over the phone. But I just plowed through them.

The waiting room was filled with patients. I found myself growing irritated. Does everyone have a 2 o'clock appointment? I wondered. But then I remembered that a lot of doctors' names were etched in the entrance door. The door to the medical area swung open and my hopes rose. But, another patient's name was called. The time was only 2:15.

Shortly after I heard, "Joanna?"

Paul and I both got up. Mary, the nurse, greeted me with a smile. She pointed to the scale, "Can you get on please?"

I was getting used to this routine. She brought us into a small room and took my blood pressure and wrote down numbers on her computer screen.

"This is your first time here?" she questioned.

"Yes."

"Dr. Heart is very nice. You'll like him."

That brought a smile to my face. "He'll be with you in a few minutes, he's just finishing up with another patient." She turned and left the room.

Paul and I looked at each other and both thought the same thing. "These people are really nice," we both agreed.

The room was tiny; there was an examining table for the patient, a chair, and a stool. Paul took the chair and I sat on the table. Within minutes, we heard a slight tap at the door and Dr. Heart walked in.

He reached out his hand and I shook it. "It's nice to meet you, Joanna."

Paul extended his hand and said, "Paul."

"Nice to meet you, Paul," Dr. Heart said. He took his spot on the stool.

He proceeded to ask me questions about my lifestyle. What did I like to do? Was I having any trouble doing any of it? Have any of my activities changed because I felt I couldn't do it?

I filled him in about my swimming and how I don't feel any different. He was clicking away on his computer but kept eye contact as much as possible. Then it was time for the stethoscope. Being nervous, my heartbeat quickened.

"Hmmm," he said. "I see why you were referred. I want to give you an echo test. Do you have time to do that today?"

I looked at Paul. I didn't know if he had plans for the afternoon. He smiled and said, "Go ahead."

"Sure," I said.

"Okay, let's do that first and then I'll talk to you about the results."

He thoroughly explained what an echo test was and his clarification put my mind at ease. No needles, just a cold disk moving around my heart area. He showed me where to wait. We sat and Paul's foot kept pace with the clock's metronome I heard in the distance.

My Lesson Learned

Put aside your companion's annoyances and focus on the fact that someone is there to share the burden.

Echocardiogram

Here I was, sitting, waiting, in a comfortable chair; the foot-tapping that is usually reserved for my husband transferred to me. Right foot over left foot, with right foot rising and falling. My husband sat next to me appearing to be engrossed in a book. He seemed to clear his throat after every page.

I heard a door open to my right and a woman, putting on her jacket on her way out, caught my eye. I knew I was up next. The door gently closed on its own. Minutes later, I heard it squeak. The technician, a cardiac sonographer, called my name, "Joanna?"

I nodded and stood up.

"I'm Doctor Kar, I'll be doing the procedure."

The word 'procedure' scared me. My heart responded by beating faster.

He moved his hand toward the door and I started to go in. Paul touched my arm, "I'll be waiting right here."

That touch released some pent-up fear.

Entering the room, I saw a screen and a keyboard which I later learned was part of the ultrasound machine. An examining table and a chair were also squeezed into this small space.

"Put your stuff here," he said pointing to the chair. Smiling, he pointed to the examining table and I obediently sat down.

"Have you ever had an echogram?" he asked.

"No," I replied as my eyes wandered around the room where I spied a clean folded paper gown waiting for me.

"This little microphone is called a transducer. I'm going to put some gel on it and move the microphone around your chest area." He looked at me and I nodded to let him know I understood.

"How long does this take?" I thought about my husband's shaking leg.

"45-60 minutes," he paused. "Have you eaten?"

He must have read my mind because I wondered about the procedure and if food would affect the results.

"No, why?"

"It doesn't matter. I didn't want you to worry if you had eaten."

Sitting down at the machine, he asked me my name and date of birth. Click, click. "I'm going to leave. If you could undress from the waist up and put this gown on. Keep the tie in the back." He got up from his chair. "I'll knock before I come in. Please face the machine."

He left and I thought about being naked from the waist up. I reflected on my mother's word when I had my first gynecology exam. "Don't be embarrassed," she had said. "When he's seen one, he's seen them all."

Before facing the machine, I took a glance at the computer screen. There was my name, Joanna Torreano, and date of birth.

I heard a gentle tapping on the door. "Ready?" he asked.

"Yes."

Settling in, he clicked a few items with the mouse. Then he put a dab of gel on the microphone and gently moved the paper gown to reveal my chest. Slowly he moved the microphone with his left hand while intermittingly clicking the mouse with his right hand. I distracted myself by staring at the nature photography on the wall behind him. Somebody thought of everything.

Then he adjusted the volume and I heard *swish, swish, swish.*

"What's that?"

"Your heart," he responded.

"Is that a good sound? I inquired.

"It's neither good or bad. It's just your heartbeat and valves opening and closing," came the non-committal answer.

How I hate not knowing yet his expertise made him aware of my results. My body, I should be in the know and I wasn't. He adjusted the paper gown to cover the area he finished scanning and moved the microphone to another area.

"We're almost done here."

I took a deep sigh.

"For this part, I'm going to ask you to take a deep breath, hold it to the count of 5. Are you ready?"

"Yes."

"Take a deep breath. Hold it. One, two, three, four, five. Breathe."

Once again the volume raised and we repeated holding my breath. *Swish, swish, swish,* and I didn't ask what the sound meant. Why bother?

"Now, that wasn't so bad, was it?" he asked.

"No," and I meant it.

Getting up, he said, "I'll leave and you can clean the gel with this," he handed me a white cloth. "When you're ready, come out and leave the door open. I'll give the results to Dr. Heart and he'll talk to you."

Getting dressed, I felt two emotions. relief in knowing my echo was done, and anxiety waiting for results.

Opening the door, Paul was in the same spot. "How'd it go?" he asked.

"There was nothing to it."

I sat down next to him and a nurse came over.

"Joanna?" she asked.

"Yes."

"Let's put you in a room. When Dr. Heart finishes with his patient, he'll see you."

We both stood up. Paul motioned for me to lead the way. We made a quick left and entered the room on the right.

"It won't be long. He's just finishing up," the nurse said before she gently shut the door.

Paul and I looked at each other. I grabbed the book I had buried in my bag and he reopened his. We both sat down and his leg began bouncing up and down.

My Lesson Learned

Waiting for results is taxing. Ignoring anxiety quirks in another is also demanding. Keeping in focus that I had companionship is critical.

1st Echo Results

Paul and I sat reading our respective books. My eyes read words, but my mind didn't comprehend any of it. Hearing doors open and close and soft voices speaking to one another became my focus. When would it be my turn?

Within a few minutes, Dr. Heart entered the room. "I took a few minutes to look at your results. He walked over to a wall chart and pointed. "See this?" he pointed to a mitral valve.

We nodded.

"Your valve is leaking a bit. I'd like to repeat the echo in six months. If there's no change, we'll just keep a watch. If there is a change, we'll talk about options. Do you have any questions?"

"I don't understand what it means."

"For now, it means nothing. But if you develop symptoms, and the valve leaks more, we'll have to figure something out."

I nodded.

"Do you have shortness of breath?"

"No."

What about when you're swimming? Any problems with chest pain?"

Another, "No."

"How about any type of exercise, any pain?"

"No."

"I have many patients with leaky valves and I just monitor them. I wouldn't worry. You have no symptoms."

His soft kind voice put me at ease. He shook our hands and led us over to scheduling.

"It was nice meeting you both. See you in six months." He walked away and I heard another patient's door open.

The lady at the desk was friendly as she scrolled the computer screen for a six-month appointment. Handing me a card with the details, she said, "Don't worry, if you misplace this, we'll call you with a reminder a few days ahead of time."

Opening the door to outside, I took a deep breath of fresh air. My feet touched the ground with a feeling of elation. But my feet were wrong.

My Lesson Learned

Being symptom-free doesn't mean you don't have an issue. It's hard to determine what normal is when you have only yourself for comparison. I thought everyone's heart banged like mine did.

Echo Testing – Six Months Later

Knowing you could have mitral valve surgery and having it are two different emotional experiences. Having a surgeon mess with your heart is frightening.

"Six months," the cardiologist said. "Come back in six months so I can compare echo-cardiogram results." I placed one foot in front of the other and didn't think about it. Why should I? I felt fine. I resumed my daily activities that included a daily one-hour walk and swimming twice a week.

I tried to keep my fear on the back burner. But the burning flame made it to the front. The more I tried to bury my anxiety, the more it blazed.

Returning from swimming, my answering machine was blinking. I pressed the message button. "This is Dr. Heart's office calling to remind you of your Friday appointment for an echo scheduled for 10:30. If you're unable to keep this appointment, please call the office at 555-5555."

Sure I thought. I'm not keeping it. I felt fine and didn't want to spend $50 for nothing.

My husband walked into the room and heard the end of the message. "You're going, right?" he said more like a statement.

"Why should I? I feel fine?"

"It's just good to get checked out," said the man who avoids all medical appointments. "I'll go with you," he said nonchalantly.

"I was thinking of canceling."

"I wish you wouldn't. I don't think that's a good idea."

"I FEEL FINE," my irritation came through.

"I think you should go," he said as he calmly walked out of the room.

I picked up my wet swimsuit and walked downstairs to hang it up. Going down the stairs, my heart was pounding. Was it from fear or was my heart misbehaving? I didn't know. I didn't want to find out either. Bits of water from the wet suit fell from my hands at the same speed as my rapidly beating heart.

Doubt filled my head, but so did dollar signs. Fifty bucks to have the cardiologist say I was fine, no thanks.

"So, what are you going to do?" my husband asked as I came back up the stairs.

"I don't know."

"Look, we have the money. It's just to check things out. I'm going to come with you. Just do it," he said with more persistence.

I didn't want to hear any bad news. If I don't go, the problem doesn't exist was my foolish train of thought. As it turned out, it was a good thing I kept the appointment. My husband was right. The echocardiogram was just the beginning.

My Lesson Learned

Just because you feel fine doesn't mean you are healthy. A $50.00 investment to your health and well-being is worth it.

2nd Echo Test

Irritated is the word I'd use to describe my feelings. Angry at my husband as he drove me to the echo test. Irked at myself for being annoyed at him when his kindness should have been my focus.

We arrived the 15 minutes ahead of schedule as requested and sat in the crowded waiting room. Paul promptly got his book and his bouncing leg commenced. I should be used to it, but I'm not.

The delay was minimal as I heard my name when the door to the office opened.

"Joanna?"

"Yes," I replied.

Paul assured me, "I'll be right here." With a pat on the shoulder, I went through the doors and into the same room I occupied six months ago. But this time, Wanda would be performing the exam. That brought comfort and I felt my shoulders relax.

"Here's the gown," she said pointing.

"I know, tie it in the back and take your top and bra off."

"Yes," Wanda said smiling.

I hoped my inward emotions of irritability didn't make it to my surface. Her kindness was genuine. I needed to relax.

"I'll be back in a few minutes and I'll knock before I come in," she said.

"Okay," and I felt a smile escape.

This isn't a big deal I convinced myself. I'm only doing this procedure because of my husband's insistence. There's nothing wrong with me. I have no symptoms. I'm only doing this for closure. I wanted to finish this chapter of my life and move on.

I heard the gentle tapping on the door.

"Come in," I said as I sat on the examining table.

Wanda asked me to lie facing her and opened my gown wide enough to get to my heart. She went through the same techniques as my previous echo. No surprises. Hearing the *swish, swish* of my valve opening and closing still frightened me. But I knew not to ask what it meant since she wouldn't tell me.

When Wanda finished the test, she asked me to open the door after I had finished dressing. She would then take me to another room to wait for Dr. Heart and the results.

"Sure, thank you," I felt more like myself.

Paul waited with me and I felt confident. No symptoms and a waste of money.

But I was about to get unexpected results.

My Lesson Learned

Stubbornness is good in some situations. When it comes to my health, I needed to lose my attitude.

Dr. Heart 2nd Echo Results

As expected, when Paul and I were lingering in the waiting room, his knee began bouncing. I tried to focus on something else. My irritation of having to take the 2nd echo and his idiosyncrasies added to my angst.

Within a few minutes, the squeak of the door alerted me to Dr. Heart's entrance. He immediately shook our hands.

"How are you feeling?" he asked.

"Great," I answered and didn't add feeling irked for spending 50 bucks for a test I didn't need.

"Any trouble swimming?"

"Nope."

"No shortness of breath?"

This was getting old. "No," I answered.

"What about chest pain?"

I really like Dr. Heart, but his digging for symptoms was giving me significant agitation.

"No chest pain," I hoped I kept my anger out of my tone.

"Well," he said with a deep sigh. "I'm going to refer you to a surgeon who deals with this part of the heart."

"Why?" I immediately questioned.

"Your results indicate that your mitral valve is unquestionably worse than it was six months ago."

My husband's active knee ceased. Although Paul's head was down in listening mode, he lifted it and said, "How much worse?"

"Six months ago, it was mild regurgitation. Now it's severe." He seemed to wait for that to register. "It's time to see a surgeon."

"What are the classifications?" Paul asked.

"Mild, moderate, severe. Six months ago, you registered as mild, you are now severe," he stated.

The room was silent. I took a deep breath, held it, and slowly let it out.

With great compassion, Dr. Heart said, "I know this is a lot to take in. Since you have no symptoms, you're going to be okay."

"Who are you sending me to?"

"Someone I'd go to if I had this condition," he answered. "This surgeon is the best. In fact, a few years back we worked together. I'd send any family member to him." He reached into a drawer and handed me a card. "Here's his name and phone number."

"Do you have any other questions?"

Paul and I shook our heads no.

"If you think of anything later, just call my office. If you have any trouble getting in to see Dr. Surgeon, call me, okay?"

"Yes," I answered.

Extending his hand, he met my eyes. "You're going to be okay, Joanna. But make and keep this appointment."

"I will," I said with conviction.

With that, he opened the examining room door and left.

Paul and I looked at each other. I grabbed his hand and we walked out together.

My Lesson Learned

Paul never said it, but I know I would have. Four words… 'I told you so.' Sometimes I wish I could be more like him minus the bouncing knee.

Dr. Surgeon Initial Call

I didn't wait long to call Dr. Surgeon's office. I came to terms that I have a problem and I needed to do something. The card with the information lay on my kitchen table. I picked it up after my morning cup of tea and figured it's time to take some action.

I dialed Dr. Surgeon's number. After four rings the message came on, 'I'm sorry, we're unable to come to the phone right now. Please leave your name, number, and a brief message and I'll get back to you as soon as possible.'

Here we go again, I thought. Leaving the requested information, I hung up and went about my day. About ten minutes later, the phone rang and a pleasant voice was on the other end.

"Good Morning, this is Joan from Dr. Surgeon's office, may I speak with Joanna?"

"Speaking," and my heart began to race.

"I was on the other line when you called. Sorry it took a bit to get back to you."

"It really didn't. It was only a few minutes," I replied.

"I understand you want to make an appointment. Can you tell me a little bit about why you need to come in?" she asked.

I filled her in about my recent echogram, the results and the referral from Dr. Heart.

"Oh, Dr. Heart, isn't he wonderful?" she said.

"Yeah, I really like him."

"He used to work with Dr. Surgeon. They're both good doctors," she spoke with confidence.

I needed to hear that. This woman made me feel comfortable. There's something to be said about having a person who lessens anxiety levels just by being kind.

She asked me a few more questions regarding medical insurance.

"Let's see," I heard clicking of the mouse. "It looks like next Thursday at 2 P.M., Doctor can see you."

"Sounds good," as I glanced at my calendar in front of me.

"Do you know where we're located?"

"Not really," and I added, "I have no sense of direction."

She patiently gave me the information.

"A few days before your appointment, I'll call to confirm. Sometimes if he gets caught up in surgery, I'll have to reschedule. That rarely happens, but I just want you to know."

"Okay."

"I look forward to meeting you Joanna. Dr. Surgeon is very competent. You're in good hands."

"That's good to hear."

"Any questions?"

I had no idea what to ask. But her warmth for me as a patient came through the phone.

"I'm good," I said. My pause was only seconds before I added, "Thank you."

"You're welcome."

When we hung up, my sensitivity to sound increased. I hadn't noticed the ticking clock in the kitchen before. There was a slight drip-drip of water that I hadn't noted until now. My whole body seemed to be susceptible to not only what was happening inside, but also outside. Tick-tock-tick-tock reminded me that the future would happen. But I wondered how much of it I'd see.

My Lesson Learned

If I ever own a business, I'd make sure the first person greeting the customer is as kind and sincere as Joan.

Dr. Surgeon Visit

I wish I could say I wasn't bothered by any of this, but that's not true. Paul, a hospital pharmacist, knew medical issues. He'd nonchalantly ask me questions throughout the day, but I wasn't fooled. He was going somewhere with his inquires, but I had no idea where. He had more experience and he was searching for my symptoms.

Getting to Dr. Surgeon's office was easy. Parking wasn't. We had to leave our car with a valet who took our key and gave us a receipt. After parking our car, he handed Paul a slip. "Hand this to someone when you're ready to get your car."

Paul thanked him and turned to me, "How I hate turning the keys over. Why can't I park my own car?"

"Yeah," was all I could muster.

The electric eye felt our presence and the glass doors opened. A police officer stood guard by the entrance. His presence compounded my fear. We were led to a receptionist.

"Can I help you?" she cheerfully asked.

"I have a 2 P.M. appointment with Dr. Surgeon," I said.

"May I see some form of ID please?"

I unzipped my purse and found my driver's license in my wallet. After handing it to her, she checked on her computer.

"There you are Joanna. 2 P.M. with Dr. Surgeon. She printed out a badge with my name and picture on it and handed it to me.

"Please wear this at all times."

Looking at Paul, she asked. "And you, sir, can I help you?"

"I'm Joanna's husband."

"No problem, can I see some ID?"

Paul dug in his pants pocket and pulled his driver's license out of his wallet. He handed it over. With a few clicks on the computer he was handed a badge with his picture and the word 'Visitor'. Mine said 'Patient'.

"Take the elevator to the third floor. Follow the sign for 'Cardiology'. Any questions?"

We looked at each other and shook our heads no.

Smiling, she said, "Have a good day." Looking to our right, she waved her hand forward and said, "Next."

I glanced at the police officer with his badge, holster, gun, and nightstick. His face seemed detached from his body. I smiled at him anyway. No response.

I hate elevators. I'm a little bit better when I have someone with me. Paul pushed the up arrow and within minutes, we walked into the metal box. The door slowly shut and I pressed the number 3. Why does everyone stare at the numbers in an elevator, I wondered.

Bing, bing, we were on floor two. Door opens. We shuffle over to let people in and out. Door closes.

Bing, floor three.

"Excuse me," Paul and I exited.

We were like mice looking for cheese. We weaved the halls together until we saw the cardiology sign. Etched in glass was Dr. Surgeon, Cardiology.

"Well, this is it," Paul said. He held the door for me.

People in their 80s and 90s shared the space. Some in wheelchairs and some with walkers nearby. *I'm 65, what was I doing here?*

With a slow gait, I made my way to the receptionist. She glanced at my badge.

"Welcome Joanna. Dr. Surgeon will be with you next."

She must have noticed my confused gaze. "There are several doctors here today."

In my state of anxiety, I hadn't noticed the other names etched in the door.

"Have a seat. Someone will be with you shortly."

I turned and saw Paul pat the chair next to him. I sat down, and grabbed a year-old magazine. Mindlessly flipping through the pages, I heard a door creak and saw a smiling face.

"Joanna?"

"Yes," I said.

"Please come in."

"Can my husband come too?" I asked.

"Of course."

Whisked into another room, we lingered in another 'waiting' room.

"I'll be right back. I need to get my stethoscope."

After she closed the door, I turned to Paul.

"I thought Dr. Surgeon was a male."

"So did I."

We later learned she was the step before the doctor. More medical questions. I should be used to it, but I wasn't. Rehashing what had occurred only brought it to the front burner. I prefer the stove being on off.

Within minutes, she returned and introduced herself.

"My name is Bridgette. I'm going to take your vitals and ask you a few questions. Then I'll bring you to Dr. Surgeon."

My blood pressure was high, no surprise there. My heartbeat elevated. Another expectation realized. She went over my medical records and confirmed my purpose for my visit.

"Yes," I assured her. My mitral valve has severe regurgitation.

Placing the stethoscope on my heart, she had me hold my breath for a count of five and then breathe.

"I can hear it," she said.

"What's it?" I asked.

"The regurgitation," she said with a smile.

I raised one eyebrow and looked at my husband.

"I have everything I need. I'll take you to Dr. Surgeon's office. It was nice meeting you."

"You too," I replied.

The door was open and we were off to receive more bad news.

My Lesson Learned

I call myself a 'closeted Christian' since I am uncomfortable around people who outwardly profess their faith. I feel like we have different Gods. Sometimes I feel like the closet is closed and I'm in there alone. Today was one of those days. Show me a sign, God, I asked.

Dr. Surgeon Consultation

"Dr. Surgeon," he said extending his hand. "Please, sit down."

There were two chairs stuffed into his small office. He pulled up my echo results on his computer.

"Let me explain everything and then I'll answer any questions you have. Okay?"

"Sure," Paul and I said in unison.

He flipped the screen toward us and began. "This is your…," and his phone rang.

"I'm sorry. I asked my secretary to put this patient through. I need to take this."

"We should leave," I said more as a statement than a question.

"No, no, please," he said moving his hand downward, "Just sit."

He picked up the phone. "Dr. Surgeon, how may I help you?"

I took a few minutes to look around the small room that overflowed with books placed every which way on a stuffed bookshelf. All publications seemed to be medically related. On the walls, various degrees and certificates relating to the heart with Dr. Surgeon's name and date of completion filled the space. It was comforting to know this guy had credentials and by the tone of his voice, a caring surgeon as he was comforting a distressed patient. I could tell by the way he reassured this individual the whole thing is routine to him. It's anything but for the people he helps.

Within minutes, he put down the phone and said, "Thank you for your patience. Now, where were we?"

With the computer screen flipped toward us, he began again.

"This is your mitral valve. As you can see, it is not fully closing like it should."

I had no idea what he was looking at. Imagine a fuzzy black and white television screen. But I remember he said to hold all questions. Didn't want to upset him.

He continued, "Blood is backing up into your lung. You don't want that. What I'm recommending is mitral valve surgery. I would go in and either repair or replace your mitral valve. After surgery, you would be in the hospital for five to seven days."

I took a deep breath and looked away from the computer screen. That can't be my heart. He must have me confused with another patient.

He continued, "If I am able to repair it, that's the best case scenario. If I have to replace it, we have two options. One is a metal valve. That will last your lifetime. But if you choose that, you will be on Coumadin for the rest of your life. If you choose, a cow valve, it will last about 20 years at tops. There will be no medications to take with that valve."

I let that sink in. I'm a no medicine-taking person. I think about whether or not I'm going to take an aspirin.

"Let's see, how old are you?" He glanced at some paperwork. "65, so at 85 you may need another surgery if you go with the cow valve. You have to think about your health at 65 and what your health may be like at 85."

He produced models from his desk. "This is what a metal valve looks like and this is a cow's valve."

I didn't want either one of them. But I didn't have a choice.

"Now, I can take your questions," he said encouragingly.

"Well, how certain are you that my mitral valve can be repaired?"

"I'm not certain at all. I won't know until I get in and look around. But if I can repair, I will repair," he said with conviction.

"Any bets on that?"

"I'm not a betting man," he replied. He sensed my hesitation. "You don't have to decide now which way you want to go. I'll have both a metal and a cow's valve available. You can tell me as late as right before surgery."

"Okay."

"How do you repair a valve?" I asked.

"It's with a needle and thread. I would stitch your valve back together again. It's a very successful surgery. I've done many of them."

"How many mitral valve surgeries have you done?" I questioned.

"Too many to count," he said with a deep sigh. "Probably thousands. I've been doing this well over 30 years. The technology has changed, but that's for the better."

He went on to explain what needed to be done before mitral valve surgery.

"Before we do anything, I need you to go for an angiogram to make sure there are no blockages. If that comes back okay, we can proceed with the mitral valve surgery. I want to be sure what I'm looking at."

"How do I schedule an angiogram?" I asked.

"Not a problem, my secretary will take care of that for you."

"You know, I just want to say that your secretary is very kind and puts me at ease."

"Yeah, she is good. We've worked together for many years. She's the best."

Looking at Paul, Dr. Surgeon asked, "Any questions?"

"No, not right now, thank you,".

"Would you like to schedule an angiogram or do you want to think about it?"

"Schedule," I said looking at Paul. He nodded in agreement.

"Okay," Dr. Surgeon said. Standing up, he continued, "Let me walk you over to Joan, she'll take it from here. It was nice meeting you both. Go home and think about the type of valve you'd like."

I wanted neither of them. But I had to make a choice.

My Lesson Learned

When I was young, my decisions seemed big, but weren't. Now that I'm older, my medical decisions are big and I wish they weren't.

Angiogram Appointment

The walk to Joan's office was a few steps, but each stride felt heavy. Being lead to a place I didn't want to be with an appointment I didn't want to make proved to be cumbersome.

But Joan was her welcoming self. Big smile on her face as she peered over her computer.

Dr. Surgeon spoke, "Joan, this is Joanna Torreano and she needs an appointment for an angiogram. Make it as soon as possible, please."

With that, he shook our hands and walked away.

I didn't like the sound of urgency in his voice, but I felt numb, desensitized to the sounds and people around me. It was as if I were walking in someone else's shoes.

"Well, it's nice to finally meet you. I know we've spoken on the phone," she said.

"Yes, and I appreciate your kindness. This is all brand new to me."

Her smile continued as she clicked the mouse searching for availability.

"Oh, I have a vacancy two weeks from today," she said looking at us for confirmation.

If I had anything on my home calendar, it didn't matter. This had to get done.

"Sure," I said.

"You have to be at the hospital at 5 A.M. to get registered. No food or water after midnight the night before the procedure. After you're finished, you will be able to eat. Any questions?

Dollar Sign Joanna showed up, "How much is this going to cost?"

A few ticks on the mouse and she answered, "Just your regular hospital co-pay."

"Is Dr. Surgeon a participating provider?"

"Yes."

I had no idea how much my co-pay was, but knew how to find the information. A simple phone call to my provider and I'd have those facts.

"Would you like me to schedule the angiogram?" she asked.

"Yes."

The mouse click to schedule lasted seconds. My angst carried on much longer. Two weeks is a long time to linger and worry.

My Lesson Learned

Keeping my mind busy helped me forget that my mitral valve would misbehave with our without my permission.

Waiting on an Angiogram

With the age of any information easily accessible, I chose to ignore any Google searching. It would have been simple to Google *'angiogram'* and learn what I would be up against. But with that comes stories from people I didn't know and I didn't want to be familiar with their experiences. In fact I told very few people I was going in for this procedure because I didn't want to hear about Aunt Betty and Uncle Fred. I already knew of a person who went in for this procedure and the next thing I knew I was speaking at her funeral. There's risk in all surgeries, and this one, had its own complications. I know people mean well, but I did the same when I was pregnant. Until it became obvious, I kept my mouth shut.

The two weeks passed slowly. I kept myself busy. I really didn't know what was going to happen. Although my husband, a pharmacist, knew, we didn't talk about it. I didn't want to know. *I don't know, is ignorance bliss?*

I set my alarm for 3:30 AM not wanting to give up my quiet time. I didn't need the buzzing reminder. I had very little sleep. I took my shower, woke my husband and we were off. We arrived before the 5 A.M. appointment time. As Paul pulled into the hospital driveway, a man seemed to appear out of nowhere, took the keys to our car, and parked it. He came back with a tag and said, "When you're ready, just give this to the valet."

I know my husband wasn't happy about turning over the keys. But he also knew how nervous I was and took this opportunity to keep his thoughts to himself.

The motion sensor for the glass door felt our presence and we were let into the hospital corridor.

An officer and receptionist chatted. I wouldn't want to converse at 5 A.M. She waved me over and the law enforcement took a slight step to the left.

"How may I help you?" she asked.

"I'm here for an angiogram," I said.

"Do you have ID please?" she questioned.

Digging in my pocket, I gave her my driver's license. Taking it, she put information into the computer.

"Oh, there you are. I see an order from Dr. Surgeon's office."

A few more clicks, she turned to another machine and out came an adhesive nametag. My picture, name, and the word Patient were printed. Handing it to me, she said, "Please have this visible at all times."

Looking at Paul, she asked. "And how may I help you?"

"I'm Joanna's husband."

"May I see some ID?"

Paul handed over his driver's license. Within minutes, he was given an adhesive nametag with his picture, name, and the word Visitor. Same instructions, "Please wear your tag where it's visible."

She pointed toward the elevators. "Take the elevator to the 4th floor. Follow the signs for angiogram." Before we left, she said, "Have a nice day."

"Really?"

My Lesson Learned

People mean well, but sometimes the wording is off.

Before Angiogram

"Good Morning Ma'am," said the cheerful aide as he greeted me before my angiogram.

What's he so chipper about, I thought to myself as I glanced at the clock that read 5:30. I noticed the room number above his head was 403.

"You're going to put on a hospital gown," he pointed to the gown hanging on the bathroom door in a plastic bag. "Then I'll be back in to take your vitals."

I looked at my husband who suddenly took a deep interest in his shoes.

The man returned. "I'm sorry," he said. "I never introduced myself. I'm Doug," he said extending his hand.

"Sir," he said talking to my husband. "I'm going to ask you to hold your wife's clothing in this plastic bag while she's in surgery. We don't want any contamination, ok?" He handed Paul the folded white plastic bag.

Paul smiled and took it.

"How long will I be gone? What's going to happen?"

"Oh, I'll be happy to answer your questions. But first, let's get you ready." He put a sheet on me and carefully smoothed it out. He then put a second sheet on me. I wondered why, but he must have read my mind.

"Contamination, best to have two sheets."

Didn't make a whole lot of sense to me, but it also didn't matter.

"Now," said Doug. "I'm going to prepare the area. I have to shave you."

Where? I thought, but didn't ask. He carefully moved the top and bottom sheet to shave off hair by my groin. Although he was very professional and made small talk to distract me, I felt embarrassed. Before I knew it, he was done.

"Now that wasn't so bad, was it?" he asked. "You had some questions for me?" Doug said.

"Yes, how long is this procedure and what are they going to do?"

"Hasn't anyone explained it to you?" he narrowed his eyes.

"No," I replied. "Just told me to come and have it done before my mitral valve surgery."

"First of all, you'll be awake."

"I don't want to be," I quickly said.

"Ma'am, have you ever had a colonoscopy?"

"Well, yes."

"Same thing, you'll be awake enough to do what they ask, but it won't hurt."

"What do you mean, do what they ask? What am I going to have to do?"

He pulled up a chair and met me eye level. "First they are going to put you in a relaxed state? Have you heard of Versed?"

"No."

Paul looked up from his shoes and chimed in, "It's a medicine that helps you relax, but you're still alert." Then Paul went back to his shoes.

"Ok, then what?" I asked.

"They are going to thread a very tiny wire to your arteries to check for any blockages. During the procedure, they will ask you to hold your breath, then exhale slowly."

"I don't know if I'll be able to follow it."

"You will Ma'am, I haven't heard of anyone who couldn't."

"Tell me about your family. Have any children?" he said by way of distracting me.

"Yes, one son, he's 32 years old. And you?"

"Two kids, a boy 14 going on 30 and a girl 16 going on 20," he said with a twinkle in his eye.

I was feeling better after having a conversation about something other than medical needs.

He turned to Paul. "Sir, while your wife is in surgery, there's coffee down the hall. Could you give me your cell phone number in case we need to locate you?"

That wasn't comforting to me. What was going to happen? Paul provided the number. I felt like a child. I wanted to ask why he'd need to contact Paul, but I didn't question him.

There was a quick knock at the door which I had no time to respond to before a nurse came in to start my IV. She came with a student nurse. The student went to my left arm.

"No one can get a line there," I said as I smiled. "Everyone always uses the right arm."

The nursing student looked at the registered nurse for advice. No words, just a quick turn of the head. "Give it a try. If you can't, then I will," she said with authority.

I wondered why my comment wasn't taken seriously. But I also realized, she's the one with the needle. I didn't want to aggravate her. After several attempts and several quietly spoken 'ouches', she gave up. The registered nurse took over. But her attempts were also unsuccessful.

"Well, I've never had this happen," said the registered nurse.

"I have," I said. "Try the right arm." I felt like I was talking to the stifling air.

"Before we do that, let me get another nurse. She can always get the needle in without any trouble," she said as she walked out the door.

That left me with the nursing student. "It's not going to work. Why is it so important that you use the left arm?"

"That's where the doctor likes it," she said, shrugging her shoulders.

Within minutes, the new nurse arrived. "So, what's seems to be the problem here?"

"I…"

The RN interrupted before I could answer.

"She claims," pointing to me, "no one can get a needle in her left arm," the RN said with confidence.

I noticed the new nurse's nametag, Beth. "Beth," I said trying to make myself visible again. I repeated the same sentence from before. "No one can ever get a line in my left arm. My right is always used."

Beth snapped the plastic gloves on her hands and placed a strong rubber band above my left elbow. Using her index finger, she felt for a vein. "Hmmm," she said. She continued to tap her finger on my arm. "Ok, let's try it now," she said with sureness. She carefully inserted the needle, but ran into the same problem.

"Ouch," I said louder than I intended.

"Oh, I see the problem. Let's give that arm a rest."

That would have worked, except there was a knock at the door. A person dressed in hospital fatigues said, "Is 403 ready for surgery?"

"In a minute," Beth answered as she scooted over to my right arm.

Yes, I thought. *Joanna* is ready. Before I was wheeled away to the operating room, Doug said, "I'll be here when you get back. See this menu," he said pointing to it. "You can get whatever you want to eat." He smiled, "The food is good here."

Food was the last thing on my mind. But his genuine concern felt good. My husband gave me a pat on my head. "See you soon, Little T."

The lady who pushed my hospital bed was dressed in a hospital gown, complete with a hair bonnet. She wasn't unfriendly, but did not attempt any small talk. She merely pushed the elevator button and we descended a few floors. More bumps, more turns, and then a right hand turn into the room. Except this was not the operating room. I had company.

My Lesson Learned

Sometimes you find compassion when you least expect it. Sometimes you have to accept that people are just doing their job. Medical staff can't be invested in every patient. The wheels on the hospital bed must keep moving.

Before Angiogram - Part 2

Hospital beds lined both sides of the wall. A nurse's aide slipped me into a vacant spot.

"Shortly, someone will be with you," said the unnamed lady who wheeled me in. "Would you like me to pull the drape?"

I looked around and quickly said, "No thanks." I saw at least four people hugging the wall in front of me. I had no idea how many were on my side except I knew there was a man. When I smiled at him, he turned away. I was hoping for some conversation. I didn't get it. Feeling scared, I started to shiver, not from cold, from nerves.

The man next to me rang for help. How come I didn't have a buzzer I wondered? A nurse came to his aid, but before she addressed his needs, she turned to me and held up her index finger. "I'll be with you in a minute."

The nurse drew the curtain and whispered voices ensued. But a curtain doesn't provide much protection. "I have to pee," I heard a soft voice. The nurse backed out of the curtain, but before she left she pointed her index finger toward me. I nodded. So, I wasn't invisible. She was busy.

When she returned, she must have handed him what he needed because I heard him relieve himself.

My curtain was closed with a quick shove of her hand. "We're really busy down here," she said by way of introduction.

"I'm Janice, I'll be your nurse," she said as she straightened up the bed sheets.

She looked at my wristband and asked me my name.

"Joanna Torreano," I replied.

"Date of birth?" she inquired.

I must have given her the correct information as she quickly moved to the computer that I hadn't noticed behind me.

"You're here for an angiogram, correct?"

"Yes."

"Well, it looks like you're next. They are just finishing up a patient." There was a slight pause and I heard some clicks on the computer. "The room needs to be cleaned and someone will come for you.

"I'll be starting an IV for fluids," she said as she quickly looked at my left arm. I noticed the glance.

"Long story, it's on my right." My irritation surfaced without my consent.

Reaching up behind me, she laid the nurse's buzzer on my lap. "Just push this," she pointed to the red button, "if you need anything." She hesitated for a second and then added, "I'll be right back to start your fluids."

If I wasn't allowed to eat or drink after midnight, why give me fluids? I didn't ask. I did hear the man next to me trying to get comfortable. The squeaking of the hospital bed along with the deep sighs wafted through the curtain. From the distance, the sound of wheels rolling on the hard white linoleum floor came closer. There was Janice with a determined walk pushing a pole with an IV bottle attached.

"This is to keep you hydrated," she said as she inserted the fluid into my PICC line.

"How long before my angiogram?" I asked.

"Shouldn't be much longer," came her non-answer. Before leaving she questioned me, "Do you need anything?"

A time for the angiogram, I thought. "No," I replied.

Filled with fluids had the expected result. Within 30 minutes, I had to use the bathroom. The nurse's call button was readily accessible on my stomach. I pushed it.

Janice was quicker than I expected at returning to me. "Can I help you?" she asked smiling. Even hurried, she was more than pleasant.

"I have to go to the bathroom. How do I do this?" I asked sheepishly.

"No problem, see the bathroom sign to your right," she said pointing to the sign. Without my glasses, I squinted. I had no idea what I was looking at. But I figured if I walked in the direction she pointed at, I'd eventually get there.

"Oh, but it's in use now," she paused. "That's okay, by time you get there, it should be available."

I wondered why a few feet should take so long. Getting out of bed wasn't an issue. Dragging an IV pole with my left hand and keeping my back end closed were the challenges. I grabbed the tie from behind with my right hand and tried to re-tie it, no luck. At that point, my modesty was leaving me. I was scared, frustrated and needed a bathroom. As I looked around the room, I saw fellow patients in the same holding pattern. Some had their eyes closed, some stared at their hands and very few smiled. Including myself, we had turned into robots. I wondered what their lives were like beyond these walls.

When I saw the restroom, I noticed a man ahead of me in line. I heard the click on the bathroom lock. The gentleman who was next moved his hand toward the bathroom, "Ladies first."

I didn't argue. "Thank you," I said re-grabbing my hospital gown from behind.

He tipped an imaginary hat.

I have a fear of elevators and being locked in a bathroom. I make it a practice to quickly lock and unlock a door before I'm seated. I noticed the puzzled look on the waiting gentleman as he saw the bathroom door open and close within seconds. There were no words in me to clarify what I was doing, so I didn't try to explain.

I made my way back to my bed, straightened out my sheets and waited.

Shortly a man in blue scrubs came to me, extended his hand, "Hi, I'm Doctor Island and I'm going to be your doctor and will be performing your angiogram. Any questions?"

"Sure, tell me what is going to happen."

He did and I learned Doug's version was very accurate.

"It should only be a few minutes. The nurses are turning the room over." He once again extended his hand, "I'll talk to you again before we get started." With a big smile, he walked away. Why was he so happy, I wondered.

I took a deep breath and listened to the silence and felt my thumping heart. Before I knew it, I was wheeled away. The angiogram was nothing like I expected.

My Lesson Learned

Being alone and not knowing what will happen next is frightening. Sometimes you just have to push through it. Hearing the beeps of the medical equipment I knew I was okay. If I stopped hearing them, there's a problem.

During Angiogram

The anesthesiologist pushed the unknown ingredients into my IV. "This is going to relax you, but you'll be able to do what we ask."

Seconds later, I heard, "Joanna?" from the same voice.

"Yes," my sleepy-self responded. I was between reality and dreaming. Lying on my back, I looked to my left and a large TV screen was looking back at me. Nearby, three women chatted about the upcoming weekend as drawers were being opened, sheets taken out, and other metal items piled up on a table on my right.

"What's going on ?" I asked to anyone who would respond. "What's all that stuff on the table?" I pointed to the growing collection.

"Oh, that's all for you," someone quickly replied.

"Why so many sheets?"

"Contamination," came the chorus reply.

Without skipping a beat, the conversation went back to weekend plans. I felt invisible. Someone fiddled with my left arm looking for a tube to put in an IV. "Other side," I said dismissively, since I felt like I didn't matter.

The doctor in blue scrubs appeared. "Dr. Island" he said. "It's time, Joanna." He asked me to look at the large screen on my left. I did, but not before noticing his slight stature and small hands.

"See this," he pointed using a cursor.

"Yes," I replied. It looked like a wire that had fallen out of its connector, just dangling.

"I'm going to feed this catheter into your arteries and ask you to hold your breath."

"Will it hurt?" I asked.

"No, you'll just feel some pressure, but nothing you can't tolerate. I'm going to inject a small amount of dye into your arteries and the dye will show if there are any blockages," he scanned the room looking at his colleagues. "I'm going to ask you to hold your breath once in a while." He paused, since he must have caught the look on my face. "Don't worry, I'll guide you."

"You'll be fine," he rubbed my shoulders. "Ready?" he turned his head. Lab coats, blue masks and gloved hands surrounded me.

I noticed an enclosed glass structure in front of me and a few people manning some type of machine. The doctor gave them a thumbs up which was returned to him. I still don't know the purpose those people served.

I felt relaxed and ready. I felt a slight pressure as the wire went up to and through my heart. I looked at the TV screen, but to me it looked like a bad black and white picture. Nothing hurt, it just felt different.

"Joanna?" I heard a voice.

"Yes," I surprised myself by responding.

"Hold your breath to the count of five when I tell you, okay? Are you ready?"

"Yes."

"Take a deep breath. Hold it. One, two, three, four, five." He counted aloud as I counted in my foggy head. "Now breathe."

I did as asked.

"You're doing great," he supported me.

I'm still amazed that I could follow his directions. Holding my breath for a few more times and watching the catheter being fed into me was mind-blowing. To me, it looked like a black and white TV picture with bad reception.

When the procedure was completed, I said, "Wow, I was awake for that whole thing."

"No, you weren't," came the immediate reply.

"Yes, I was," I quickly replied. But then realized I never saw the catheter removed.

"You think you were, but you weren't."

Intentionally, I closed my eyes. I shut my mouth. Why argue?

"I'll be up to talk to you and your husband in 20 minutes."

I opened my eyes in time to see him remove his facemask. He gently patted my right arm. "See you soon." After a quick glance at my chart he added, "Joanna."

My Lesson Learned

The angiogram procedure was painless. The anxiety leading up to it, wasn't. Maybe I should have Googled it so I'd be a more informed patient.

After the Angiogram

"She's coming around," I heard the same voice that I had heard while waiting for the angiogram.

Opening my eyes, my husband and Doug, the medical aide, stood by my side.

"How are you Little T?" my husband asked.

"What did they find out?" I immediately asked.

Doug jumped in. "Oh, we'll know in a bit."

"Dr. Island told me he would come up and talk to me," I said.

"Oh, that doesn't usually happen," Doug sounded sure of himself.

"But he promised," I felt like a whiny five-year-old.

"Well, we'll just have to wait and see." Changing the subject, Doug handed me a menu. "This is the great food I told you about. Order whatever you like. But you must stay on your back for a few hours. By then, it'll be lunch time and you can eat."

I looked at my husband who rarely sits still. His leg bounced up and down as he turned the pages in his book.

I fell asleep. The next thing I knew, there was a knock at the door. Dr. Island was at my bedside. Paul put down his book and my ears perked up.

"Everything looks good, no blockages," he said with a smile.

I exhaled deeply. Another deep breath come out of my husband.

"I'll get these results to your cardiologist, Dr. Heart. Make an appointment to see what the next step is, okay? Any questions?"

My husband and I both answered in unison. "No."

Before leaving, Dr. Island shook our hands.

I knew he'd come and talk to me. He promised and one thing I'm good at is measuring a person's integrity. I was right.

The food was as good as Doug had assured me it would be. But my appetite took a beating from stress.

Putting my street clothes back on, I thanked Doug for his excellent care, grabbed my husband's hand and we walked down the hall. Paul pressed the elevator button for floor one. The door slammed shut. This time I didn't mind getting in the metal box. I put this ordeal behind me.

My Lesson Learned

You can discover kindness in unexpected places. But sometimes you have to look for it.

Phone Call to Dr. Surgeon

Since I received clearance that I had no blockages, I was able to schedule mitral valve surgery.

Dr. Surgeon's receptionist, Joan answered the phone. Although making appointments is routine for Joan, it's anything but for the caller. However, Joan's genuine warmth came through the phone.

No waiting and a person picked up.

"Dr. Surgeon's office, how may I help you?"

"This is Joanna Torreano and I need to schedule mitral valve surgery."

"Oh, hi, Joanna. Your results came back okay?" she questioned.

"Yes," I answered.

"Let me take a look. I'll put you on hold."

Soft music came through the phone. How would she know I told the truth without checking? I took the opportunity to grab my calendar. The music ended. Joan's voice came back on the line.

"Your angiogram results are here. Everything looks good. Let's see what I can do about scheduling."

I imagined her computer mouse searching for dates. "How's April 24th?"

Flipping my calendar to the next month, April 24th was empty.

"Looks good here," I said.

"Where are you having your pre-surgery tests done?" she asked.

"What pre-surgery tests?" I questioned. "I didn't know I had to do anything."

"Oh, yes, it's mandatory," came the response.

"What do I need to do?"

"You'll need an electrocardiogram, a chest x-ray, and a blood test at least two weeks before surgery."

"How do I do that?"

"You can get a script here or go to your primary doctor," she offered.

"Makes sense to have you do it," I said.

"Sure. Where would you like it done?"

"Where do most people go?" I asked.

"Most people come here, Heart-Vascular Hospital, so everything is in one spot."

"Let's do it then."

She gave me an appointment two weeks prior to April 24th. After going for my pre-surgery tests, I thought I was set.

But on the day of surgery, with just a sheet covering me, I was in for another surprise. My test results had gone missing.

My Lesson Learned

I should have had a hard copy of my pre-surgery tests with me on the day of surgery. If I was on meds, I would have brought a list of medications.

Admission - Part 1

April 24, 2017 came whether I wanted it to or not. I set my alarm for 3 o'clock but didn't need the shrill sound to waken me. My eyes looked around my bedroom and focused on the photo I treasured. It is a grandmother sitting in a prayerful position. Hope she says a few for me, I thought. I had dreaded the day too long. Now it was time to just get it over with. Paul and I drove to Heart-Vascular Hospital in Buffalo, New York, in silence. The roads were not congested. The sound of the tires hitting the pavement was the only noise that filled the car's interior. We were told, "Be here at 5:30 A.M. for your 7:30 surgery."

I didn't know what type of surgery I was getting. Would it be a mitral valve repair or a replacement? It was up to the doctor after going in and seeing what the damage required. I remember the doctor's words, "I'll know once I get in there."

The sound of tires hitting the dry pavement continued to fill the car's interior. Fast-food billboards beckoning passersby for breakfast specials reminded me of my hunger. "No eating or drinking after midnight," I had been told.

My mind wandered back to a few nights ago. I had gotten my affairs in order. Paul does little with our finances so I wrote everything down. Many times I tried to show him the information, but he dismissed me.

"I don't need it," he waved his hand in a halting position.

As we approached April 24th, I became more persistent.

"Okay, Okay, he said. "Show me." His agreement didn't bring me comfort. It brought fear.

We arrived at the hospital to the circular driveway where we were told an attendant would take our car. True to the secretary's word, a man approached us and said, "Good Morning, if you don't mind, I'll take your car and give you a paper detailing where you can find it," he said with a smile. With the car door open, the crisp air brought a shiver to my already uptight body.

Paul handed over the keys. After the attendant was out of earshot, Paul said, "I hate this. Why can't I park my own car?"

"Yeah," I responded with thoughts far away.

The valet returned with the receipt. The hospital door sensor must have felt our presence as the entrance automatically opened. I felt swallowed up as we walked in to a very empty lobby. Tall ceiling, fluorescent lights, and a lady sitting behind a desk with an armed police officer by her side. Having law enforcement present elevated my anxiety, not reduced it.

"Good Morning," she said in a chipper voice.

I barely smiled.

"How may I help you?" she asked.

"I'm here for surgery."

"Name, and some ID please?"

After a few clicks on the computer, she said, "Uh huh, there you are. You are scheduled for mitral valve surgery, correct?"

"Yes, " I replied.

After a few seconds and the sound of a printer working, she handed me my badge with my name and the word 'Patient'.

"Please wear this at all times."

She turned to Paul, "And you sir, why are you here?"

"I'm her husband," he politely replied.

"May I have some ID?" Paul handed over his driver's license. She put it through a machine and it printed a badge that showed 'Visitor' with his picture.

"There you go, wear this at all times," handing a badge to him. Although she was smiling, I had a difficult time matching her grin. "Your next step is right around the corner," she said pointing to the right. "That's where you will get registered. Any questions?"

None other than I thought she just registered me. We were on our way. I didn't know then how many mandated procedures I would encounter.

My Lesson Learned

Unfamiliar circumstances can be very intimidating. I learned I had to swim through them to the other side letting the splashes and waves seek their own destination.

Admission - Part 2

We walked into the appropriately-named waiting area. We were in delay mode. We were the only people around in this dark room. I sat on the hard chair. My mind was shutting down. There was nothing but a black blank screen in my head. In a few seconds, the lights in a distant room went on, however, my mind was still empty.

I hugged my stomach as it growled from lack of food. Despite the warm temperature, my body was shivering from anxiety.

I leaned over to Paul hearing the sound of rattling keys fill my ears. "Seems like someone is here," I spoke in a soft voice.

"Yeah, it does, doesn't it?" was his whispered response. I could smell the orange flavored candy on his breath. After placing it in his mouth, he apologized, "Sorry, I forgot you can't eat."

I just nodded. We all handle stress in different ways.

Within a few minutes, a woman popped her head out of an adjoining room.

"May I help you?"

I wondered if she could relieve my anxiety or the stress headache that was poking through like needles in a pincushion.

We walked over and I handed her the paperwork we were given. "I guess you need this," I said. *Was the paper shaking on its own or was my hand contributing to the quivering?*

"Thank you, I do." She motioned toward her room and we obediently followed. I spotted another hard chair. My body was getting use to the stiffness of the chair as well as the rigidity of the situation.

"Do you have your insurance card with you?" she asked as she booted up her computer. What sounded like tired beeps filled the air. They matched my fatigue.

I dug the card out of my pants pocket and handed it to her. She swiped my card through a machine and handed it back. She adjusted her eyeglasses as she looked over the paperwork. This lady was efficient, but I needed a caring touch. I could tell, I wasn't going to get it. "Everything looks good, I just have to print out your admissions paper that you'll give to the people on the floor." She stood up quickly, turned her back and walked out. While she was gone, my husband and I sat saying nothing to each other. We seem to react to pressure in the same way. A few minutes later, she returned with my paperwork.

"Please sign here," she said fingering the bottom of the paper. Pointing she said, "You will go out this door, turn right, and take the elevators to the fifth floor. Once you get there, they will explain what you are to do next." She stood up letting us know her job was over.

All I could do was nod in recognition that I understood her directions, but I really didn't. Her lips were moving, but my brain was as dark as the walls that enveloped me.

Paul waited for me to leave the room first. I looked left and right for an elevator. I was in robotic mode. Without a word, Paul pointed to the right. I walked over and pushed the up arrow key. It felt sticky. The elevator door opened and we stepped in. The sound of the reverberating shutting door went through me but not before the hospital smells seeped through.

On the fifth floor, the staff was hustling around and barely noticed us. My brain kicked in and pushed me to make myself visible. I walked up to someone who appeared to be in charge and asked, "Excuse me, where do I go? What am I supposed to do?"

The harried response was, "Please wait over there," a nurse said pointing. "We'll be with you in a few minutes."

I looked at Paul for some reassurance. He shrugged his shoulders and gently placed his comforting hand on my back as he led me to another hard stiff chair.

My Lesson Learned

I felt like I was shoved from bench to bench. Other people's needs are as important as mine. It's difficult to take a back seat, especially when the bench is hard.

Hospital Procedures

I moved around on the hard bench due to nerves. I couldn't get comfortable. What seemed like hours later, but was probably minutes, a nurse came.

"My name is Gina and I will be taking care of you. What is your name?" she asked holding a clipboard full of papers.

"Joanna Torreano," I replied.

She used her pen and made a checkmark on her paper.

"Date of birth?"

I responded and saw another checkmark being made.

This time she looked up and smiled. "Let's go this way, please." She pointed down the hall. Paul and I both shot up. She turned to my husband, "Not you, sir, I'll call you when she's ready."

Paul looked at me helplessly and slowly sat back down, but not before a slight touch on my back. The nurse turned to him and said, "It'll be a few minutes. There's coffee over there." What he didn't need was caffeine to heighten his existing nervous jitters.

The room we entered did not look like a typical hospital room. There was a reason for that. It wasn't. It was a place where I had more mandated procedures. I took a seat on a high-backed chair that reclined. The nurse smiled and looked at her clipboard, removed the top sheet and began her questions.

"Name?"

I thought, but didn't say, it hasn't changed since our walk down the hall. My stress level and irritation grew as the questions that she had just asked me were repeated again. Then it was time for the blood-pressure cup and no surprise, my blood-pressure was elevated.

"Ok, it's time for a shower," she said pointing to the stall in the right-hand corner.

"I took one an hour ago with the mandated soap," I said trying to curb back my irritation.

"Hospital procedures. You need to take one here. We need sterile conditions in the operating room."

Before I had time to protest, and without any further discussion, she handed me a bag for my contaminated clothes and handed me a plastic-wrapped hospital gown.

"Tie the gown in the back," she explained.

I stepped into the shower and had half a mind of just running the water and opening the bar of soap. But instead I turned on the faucet and quickly warm water sprayed down. The bath soap, which was the same soap I had just used at home, was in a plastic seal. I broke it open and used it once again. There was no lather, it felt like I was spreading flour all over my body.

Next came the breaking of the seal of the wrapped towel. I dried off and placed the used towel on the ground as instructed. I felt like a slob just throwing the towel on the floor, but hey, hospital procedures. I opened the door and found my husband and Gina waiting and making small talk. They looked like they were having a wonderful time together just chatting. Normally I'd be happy about that, but not today, I was annoyed.

"They're ready for you," Gina said. Before I could react, I was sitting in a wheelchair. I wondered if it had been sterilized, but didn't ask. I was pushed to my next destination. Paul ambled along behind, carrying the bag of my contaminated clothing.

My Lesson Learned

I learned when you have little power and you're being asked to comply with mandated procedures, it's best to shut up and obey. But it's a good idea to have an advocate if things get out of hand.

Holding

The staff wheeled me into a room with only a white sheet covering my gowned body. My dry skin felt scratchy next to the cotton cloth. The sheet was up to my neck and I was up to my collar in worry. A lady in blue scrubs identified herself as Mary. She came up to me and asked my name and why I was in the hospital. In my head, I thought, don't you know. But I promptly replied, "Joanna Torreano, mitral valve repair or replacement." I think this is one of their mandated procedures, making sure the right person with the correct surgery.

Hearing click, click, from the computer, I must have matched her information.

"The anesthesiologist will be here shortly and give you something to relax you," she said smiling. "Are you warm enough?"

"No, I'm freezing," I said as my body started to shiver.

"Yeah, we have to keep it cool in here because of all the medical equipment. Don't want them to overheat." Before walking away, she turned and spoke over her shoulder, "I'll be right back with a warm blanket."

While she was gone, I had the white ceiling and the humming lights to keep me company. The voices in the background seemed to fade and became muffled like children whispering in a friend's ear. My fingers began tapping under the sheet as though I was just learning to play the piano and hitting all the wrong notes.

The lady in blue scrubs returned and carefully placed the warm blanket over me.

"Better?" she said smiling.

"Much better," I said.

Hushed voices all around asking people their names and purpose of hospital stay. 'Click, click' of the computer mouse hit my ears reminding me of the sound of hail falling from the sky.

Soon, a woman in a white coat approached me. She was professional, but her commanding mannerisms let me know she had a job to do.

Once again, I was asked, "Name?"

"Joanna Torreano."

'Click,' another piece of hail hit my ears.

I heard the scrolling of the mouse.

"Hmmm," she said looking perplexed. "Where did you have your pre-surgery tests completed?"

"Here," I said feeling my panic rise.

Another hum and the sound of the mouse scurrying for cheese across the computer screen.

"How long ago was that?" she asked without looking at me and adjusting her glasses as she continued to scroll. I detected a slight scent of lemon perfume when she readjusted the sleeve of her lab coat.

"I was told it had to be two weeks prior to surgery. I don't remember the exact date," I replied as my heartbeat louder as if to chime into the answer.

"I'll be right back," she said. Before she left, she quickly added, "Don't worry, I'll find the results."

My warm blanketed body responded with this information by doing a shake of its own. My toes cramped up like an orange being squeezed for juice. A nurse, having overheard the conversation, quickly came over and put her hand on my arm. "Don't worry. This happens all the time," she placed a strong emphasis on *all.* "And," she continued, "She always finds the results."

My heart must have been listening as it slowed its drumbeat. My toes responded by relaxing.

About ten minutes later, the anesthesiologist returned, quickly glanced at me, "No, problem, I found the test results." She resumed her computer clicking. Turning to me, she said, "I'm going to give you something for relaxation. You will be alert to answer any questions, but more relaxed than you are now."

Before I knew it, she had a syringe in her right hand that she had pulled out of her front pocket. It was like a bad horror movie with the smile she gave me before pushing the contents of the syringe into my body.

Next thing I knew I felt swallowed up like I was swimming underwater with only a small chance of surfacing for air.

My Lesson Learned

Keep dates of pre-screening tests in your head. Or better yet, have your loved one keep a hard copy so you can refer the anesthesiologist to that person.

Roll-'Er-In

True to the anesthesiologist's comment, I could respond to the people around me. But I didn't feel like talking. I felt like it was two in the morning; groggy, but aware. Someone wheeled me from the waiting area into the operating room. The jostling of the wheels underneath me shook my senses awake.

When I arrived my words came alive. "Where's the person who is putting my heart on a machine?"

I saw a hand raise behind one of several apparatuses.

"Keep me alive," I blurted out.

The heart team's perfusionist, the medical technician who controlled the heart machine, smiled, "I will," he said adding a thumbs up.

Being aware of what was going on brought me no comfort. To the right of me I saw piles of sealed instruments. People in scrubs talked about their weekend plans. Normal for them and normal for me were different. I caught the eye of a nurse. "What's all that for?" pointing to the pile on my right.

"That's all for you," she said.

"For what?" as she continued putting plastic bags in various piles. She looked at tags before deciding where she would heap it.

"For your surgery, you'll use all of this," she replied.

"All set?" she said turning to her fellow scrub-mates.

As if on cue, they gathered around me. One on my right side, one on my left and someone at the foot of the operating table. They snapped on plastic gloves and someone kicked a metal garbage can my way. I heard the ripping of plastic and was covered with a cloth. Second sheet, same thing. The material unfolded much like a flag is folded at a funeral.

"Why two sheets?" my groggy-self asked.

"Contamination," came the chorus response.

They must have had enough of me because a person with a syringe appeared.

"We're almost ready to begin. I'm giving you something to relax." She pushed the ingredients from the needle into my IV. My body felt warm and tingly.

No more voices, no more questions. The next thing I knew I woke up in ICU.

My Lesson Learned

Had I kept my mouth shut, I may have been awake for the pre-surgery routines. If I want to know what's going on, I shouldn't ask too many questions. They have the 'relaxing' medication.

ICU - Part 1

I wanted to check in with myself to see if I was still alive. I enjoyed the stillness around me. Close by I heard, "She's coming around. I think she's awake."

I opened my eyes and a blood pressure cuff was being pumped on my upper arm and a smiling nurse looked at me. I glanced at the clock, 6:45. I looked out the window. It was getting dark. Was this the next morning or was I in surgery since 7:30 A.M.? I wondered and finally asked.

"No," she replied. "You were in recovery. Your husband wanted me to tell you he left half an hour ago."

I nodded.

She continued, "Something about having to get the dogs out."

Another nod and I closed my eyes soaking in the stillness. I heard the Velcro separating as the blood pressure cuff was removed. The sound startled me. But not enough to keep me awake. The next thing I knew my blood pressure was being taken by a new nurse. The clock read 6. I wasn't sure if it was morning or night. Beside losing myself, I was losing track of time.

"Let's see how you're doing?" she said as she looked at my right breast.

Nothing could prepare me for the sight. "How come it's so big and bruised?" I asked.

I wondered how I was going to wear a bra with one B breast and one D breast. I had a solution, no bra. I don't need it.

"Oh, that's where the doctor went in to reach your mitral valve." She poked at my breast. "But everything looks good, no sign of infection," she said smiling.

"Was the mitral valve repaired or replaced?" I asked.

A few clicks on the computer screen and she replied, "Repaired."

Good, I thought, no long term meds.

Being in ICU is both comforting and frightening. I was well taken care of, but worried about the close monitoring. I was told I would be out in seven days, but had no knowledge of an ICU stopover.

I felt physically uncomfortable. I had tubes everywhere. One to eliminate urine. I learned later I had a tube to eliminate liquid around my lung. Another tube was down my throat and oxygen was pumped in my nose. I didn't expect any of this. It frightened me. My movement was limited, but I didn't think about it. I didn't leave my bed for 2 days. Everything was automated, including my food. Drip, drip, drip.

Although I had a tube down my throat, I was surprised that I could talk. But I didn't feel like it. I remember asking the surgeon before surgery when I could go back to swimming. He had replied, "You're not going to feel like it for a few months." In my head, I thought he was wrong. But knowing how I felt at that moment, I wasn't sure I ever wanted to crawl out of bed. It didn't matter. They weren't going to let me.

My Lesson Learned

Although I feel I'm an independent woman, sometimes you have to relinquish the title and become dependent.

ICU - Part 2

"I'm going to take out the tube down your throat. It won't hurt, but it will be uncomfortable." The PA (Physician's Assistant) stood over me and continued. "Take a deep breath. Hold it and slowly let it out."

I surprised myself that I could follow the directions. My brain felt foggy due to the anesthesia. The PA was right. Removing the tube didn't hurt. I could breathe again. I hadn't realized how constricted my breathing had been. I was shocked at the length of the tube stuffed down my throat.

"I'll come back and take the tube out of your right lung," she paused, "in a bit."

I didn't know I had a tube in my right lung. I did know nurses would pick up a plastic bag on my right side and write down liquid measurements. But I had no idea where the tube was attached nor did I think to ask. Being in ICU is a numbing experience.

While in ICU, I slept. I had no concept of time. There was a clock straight ahead of me, but I didn't know if it was day or night. I was fed by a drip attached to a long pole. There were other ingredients being pumped into me too. My husband, being a pharmacist, occasionally walked over to read labels.

"Everything looks good," my husband said after reading the labels. "This bag is Dextrose, your food." Moving to the next bag, he said, "This is Dilaudid, a painkiller."

"I'm not in any pain, why am I on that?"

His next comment had us both laughing. "You're not in any pain *because* of the medication."

"I don't want it!" I said forcefully.

"Okay, but you're not going to want the pain either."

Closing my eyes, I pondered his statement. Sheepishly I said, "I'll keep it."

If my husband wasn't a pharmacist, how would I know what was being pumped into me? Would I be as complacent as I was and not ask questions? Why wasn't I advocating for myself? I still don't know the answers to my own questions.

My Lesson Learned

It was good to have someone with me who is an advocate. Meds mess with my head.

Doctor Visit

From the corner of my eye, I noticed the doctor who did my surgery coming my way. Surrounded by several people with tired eyes and clipboards, these men and women wearing white lab coats fenced me in. By way of introduction, Dr. Surgeon said, "These people are students. Are you okay with them being here?"

I wouldn't have said no, but it would have been nice to have a heads up.

"How are you feeling?" he asked.

"I'm tired," I responded.

"That's normal," he said reassuringly. He jotted something down in his notebook. I felt like Elaine Benes in the Seinfeld episode when she wondered what the doctor was writing about her.

"From now on, you'll be seen by my assistant. If there are any problems, she'll contact me," he paused. "I don't expect any."

With that, he left as quickly as he came in. It was like a visit from a friend who didn't want to stay long. He didn't listen to my heart. I assumed he read the notes from the many nurses who have been in and out of the room. I didn't think to question him and probably wouldn't have if the thought had occurred to me. I was slowly losing myself in the ICU.

Before surgery, he thoroughly went over the procedure and patiently answered any questions I had. I know he was busy, but I needed a little more mothering. But he was on to his next patient.

I was left frightened and relieved. Thankful I was alive; scared by all the connections I had to various medical machines.

Why was dinner ice chips? When would I have real food? Would this exhaustion ever leave me? So many questions swirled around my head. Before I knew it, I was sound asleep again.

My Lesson Learned

Being in ICU caused me to pause. During the downtime, I realized I wasn't afraid to die. I felt at peace and I wish I knew why.

Helplessness

Being totally dependent on another person to do everything made me feel stranded. The emotional island I was on was self-made. Although there were people around, I couldn't feel their presence. My body and mind were shutting down.

When I was in ICU, the ratio of nurse to patients was two to one. Wires and tubes were attached to various parts of my body. Although I was in ICU for two days, the faces of the nurses changed every 12 hours. The consistency was that there wasn't any. I was given help to maintain this medically induced existence. What struck me was I didn't care. An eerie peacefulness flooded me. My fate was in someone's else's hands and I accepted it.

When I was vertical, I led a purposeful life. As a reading teacher, I had had daily interactions with children and adults. The 'aha' moment does exist and I was fortunate to witness the twinkle in children's eyes when they understood how to decode written language.

Now I was horizontal with only the white ceiling to keep me company. Daily, someone would bathe me. One aide gently washed between each toe and slowly rubbed the bottom of my feet. To me, it was as if she was willing life back into my body. I remember her tenderness, but can't forget the fact that my feet were going nowhere. Human touch brought me back to reality, if only for a temporary reprieve. For a short time, I felt like I was more than tubes and wires.

All I was doing on my own was breathing. Even with that I had help. I had a nasal cannula that provided oxygen at a steady rate.

When strangers cleaned my body, some talked: some remained silent, I don't know which is better.

I knew that dying was a possibility, but I felt peaceful with that realization: the beeping sounds would stop. I would be transported to the next gathering place. Having no fight, I didn't recognize myself.

I didn't want to leave this world, but I had had a good life. Teaching was my passion, never a job. I knew I was one of the lucky ones.

Now in ICU, I was like a flat tire with a deep nail and a locked steering wheel. There was no AAA to call.

My Lesson Learned

I had taken for granted trips to the grocery store and lunch with friends. When my every move was monitored, I realized how much I had taken for granted. It's true, you don't know what you have until it's gone.

Regular Room

Being wheeled into a regular room after ICU made me nervous. The excellent care I got from the Intensive Care nurses was going to be replaced. What kind of attention would I be getting as one of several patients?

Being drugged for pain, I wasn't sure if I caught a uniformed officer passing my door or if I imagined it. He was probably off duty and visiting someone, I rationalized.

The bed had buttons to push to change my position. I put it in the seating point. Everything felt uncomfortable. I filled my time sleeping. I couldn't get comfortable since I feared pulling out anything that was keeping me together. My daily stretching routine stopped. Who knows what I would have pulled away from myself?

Laying in bed, feeling helpless and being totally dependent on others isn't enjoyable. I had time on my hands and went to visit the thoughts in my head. I should never have gone alone. The space was fully occupied with fear. I squeezed myself in anyway, but panic overpowered me. I quickly left and returned to the reality of my hospital bed.

A nurse appeared and her presence brought me back to my truth.

"Joanna," she said smiling. "If you need anything, just push this red button," she said pointing to the call button on the bed.

I smiled.

"Okay, now we're going to get you up to sit on the chair. Ready?"

No, I thought, "Yes."

"Use the walker," she said as she placed it to the side of the bed. "Let me show you how." She demonstrated how to swing my legs over, grab the handles and use the strength in my arms to pull myself up. She made it look easier than what it was for me.

The nurse must have read my mind. "It's normal to feel your heart race. You've been in bed for 2 days."

With her reassurance, I felt myself relax and my heart rate slowed.

Carefully I swung my legs over and planted them on the floor. The chair, only a few feet away, looked further than it was.

"Come on, you can do this. I'm right here," the kind nurse said.

"I'm feeling light-headed."

"Take your time. I'm not going anywhere." I noticed the hustle-bustle outside my hospital room.

I took a deep breath and attempted to use the walker. I was successful and six steps later, I flopped into the chair exhausted.

"Now, remember, don't get up unless you call for help," she said deliberately. Before leaving, she turned on the TV and handed me the remote.

"What would you like to watch?" She lowered the volume on The Price is Right.

I heard the ding-ding-ding getting softer and saw a smile on the contestant's face since she was closest to the retail value.

"That channel is fine," acting more interested than I felt. I didn't want the TV. I didn't want her. I needed time to process the fact that I had heart surgery.

"Oh, before I leave, " she handed me a heart pillow. "Use this, like this," she pressed the pillow next to her heart, "if you need to cough."

"Why the pillow?"

"It won't hurt as much."

It didn't make any sense to me then and doesn't present any logic now. But she was right and the pillow became my Linus blanket.

The nurses' station was right outside my door. I heard the beeps come through as other patients requested help. The squeaking of a swiveling chair and the footsteps of a nurse were part of my daily sounds.

I didn't want to bother any of the nurses when I needed to go to the bathroom. I didn't want to ask for help to get back in bed. I'm an independent woman out of the hospital and I was determined to be one in the hospital. However, medical personnel had other thoughts. I had to go to the bathroom, so I cautiously pulled myself up and stood up. "Not bad, " I thought to myself. I took a few steps and noted the proximity of the bed should I need to fall into it. It didn't matter, a nurse bolted through my door.

"WHAT are you doing?" she asked.

"Going to the bathroom," I replied as loudly as her question was.

"I told you, not to do anything unless we were with you," she said with more kindness.

I matched her tone. "I know, but you're busy and I can do this."

"Not yet. Not until you're cleared," she paused as if gathering her thoughts. "You just had heart surgery."

"It was only a repair."

She repeated, "You just had heart surgery."

She walked me to the bathroom and waited outside the door. Instead of going back to the chair, I went to the bed.

"I'm tired, I want to sleep."

Graciously, she helped me into bed. But before she left, she gave me some unwanted words. "Don't get out of bed on your own. Use your call button," she said pointing to the button she had replaced on my bed.

With that, she left and the drone of the TV put me to sleep. I went into blissful rest, but I made more mistakes during my stay.

I learned to use my call button. But at night, I learned some of the nurses were coming from homes with small children. They were exhausted. I made a point of asking about their families. I wanted to know them as people. But knowing their backgrounds also caused me to sparingly use my call button.

Unfortunately I was given Lasix, a drug that helps you eliminate liquids. Bottom line, I had to pee a lot. I held it as long as I could. But it was time to use the call button.

I met Annie, a nurse with two small children, the night before. She was back.

"Yes," she said pleasantly.

"I have to use the bathroom."

"No problem."

I got out of bed and walked to the bathroom under her watchful eye. To make conversation, I said, "I remember you told me about your kids. Get any sleep?"

She laughed, "Yeah, my mom took them so I could rest. I'm feeling good."

Reaching the bathroom door, I pulled the handle and noticed it opened the wrong way.

Annie shook her head, "Yeah, I know, it's backwards, it's not you."

The bathroom was very clean. The pull cord should I need it was right by the toilet. I hadn't noticed it before. The toilet had an insert that I never saw before. I relieved myself and before flushing I dumped the urine from the collection pan.

Opening the door, Annie was calmly waiting and watched me make my way back to bed. Before leaving my room, she walked into the bathroom. I thought that was odd. I quickly found out why she went in.

"Why did you flush the toilet?" she asked

Flabbergasted, I replied, "Why wouldn't I?"

"You're on Lasix and we're measuring your input and output."

"You are? I didn't know that."

"That pan inside the toilet is a specimen collection pan. We need to know if we have to increase or decrease your Lasix."

"That's news to me," I replied.

"I thought you knew. Sorry. Just leave the urine and we'll document it and dump it."

Falling back to sleep, another unexpected person arrived at my door.

"Time to go for a walk," the chipper Physical Therapist announced as he came into my room. "My name is Jim."

"I'm not ready for that yet," I said with more calm than I felt.

"You'll be fine," he said as he placed the walker in front of my chair.

"Place your hands on the seat like this." He positioned his hands.

I did as he asked.

"Now, press down with your hands and use your arms to help you stand."

First try, I rose a couple of inches and fell down.

"Push harder, you can do it."

Second try, I got up but felt wobbly. He must have read my mind.

"It's normal to feel shaky. You've been in bed for two days," he said encouragingly.

Use it or lose it, immediately came to my mind.

The walker had wheels that seemed to move independently of my decision. I had to learn to take control. My self-confidence took a hit. I couldn't even manage a walker.

Moving slowly, Jim and I meandered the hall. When feeling a pinch in the heart area, I panicked, but kept it to myself. The rolling walker seemed to calm me down and my maneuvering became a little bit more leisurely. I walked for about five minutes and became winded. My heart was beating faster than it had during my lounging time.

"Ready to go back?" Jim asked.

"Yes," I said, but I hoped for more stamina.

Walking the hall I saw two police officers and a person dressed in the same hospital gown I wore. The officers were on each side of the patient. The officers' attire consisted of badge, uniform, gun, and a stick.

I then realized, the person in the room next to me is a prisoner. We were walking toward one another. I caught his eye. "Good morning," I said. He barely looked at me. He may have given me a quick smile. The police officers straightened their backs.

When did kindness become a threat I wondered?

I went to my room as he was escorted to his area.

Jim didn't mention what had just occurred and neither did I. "I'll be back tomorrow. We'll walk further."

I collapsed in my chair as I heard the prisoner's door next to me close. But I felt like the hostage.

My appreciation for the human body was growing faster and faster. I took care of my body pre-surgery. Being careful of what I ate and exercising regularly was part of my daily routine. But I never thought about the different organs and the functions they perform.

I hadn't realized that when they poured water in my bedside pitcher they were monitoring how much I drank. I remember seeing an aide pour some water and write something down. I had no idea what she was writing. But now I did.

The hard work nurses do daily and cheerfully surprised me, especially when I learned some of them completed a 12-hour day.

"How do you work 12 hours and stay alert?" I inquired one day.

The answer I got from everyone, "Oh, you just get used to it."

My strength came back slowly during my hospital stay. The careful monitoring of everything I did was needed. I didn't like it then, but it was vital that I followed instructions. Like I used to tell my students, *'Don't be a rule breaker'*. I should have heeded my own advice.

My Lesson Learned

Hospital procedures are there for a reason. Nurses are overworked and tired. I could be an obedient patient or contrary. I needed to be compliant.

Visitors

Before going into the hospital, I repeatedly told both family and friends, "Don't come and see me. I'll be sick and don't want company."

My request was not honored. In fact, my niece sheepishly knocked on the hospital door and said, "Josie, are you going to kick me out?"

My son walked in behind her carrying my robe that I asked for from home. They didn't stay long, but did bring laughter into the room.

As a child, anytime a friend or family member was hospitalized, we piled into our car and visited the afflicted. I always thought that was inconsiderate. But my parents had other ideas. "It shows you care, Joanna." I thought differently and didn't want my surgery to be a gathering place for family.

When my priest asked me where my surgery was, I told her, "Don't come, call if you want, but don't come."

After four days in the hospital, my phone rang. It was my Pastor. "I won't come, but I did call." It was nice talking to her and knowing that someone was thinking of me.

Another knock at the door and my brother walked in. "I know you said no visitors, but I'm your brother and I won't stay long." He honored his word. It was good to see him, but my eyes fought to stay open.

The days spent in the hospital were not restful. My blood pressure was taken in a non-routine manner. Being near the nurses' station brought the constant sounds of beeps, which became my new existence. No silence, not even at night. Since I could hear the beeps, it reaffirmed that I was still alive.

Thinking back, I'm not sorry I requested no visitors. I'm also glad they didn't listen.

My Lesson Learned

It gets lonely being in a sterile environment where everything is monitored. Having family break up the monotony helped with the boredom.

From Nun to Married

It's been said the first step is always the toughest. My experience is the second, third, and fourth were equally difficult. I had never used a walker. When I took my first step, the wheels propelled me further than I expected. Just another experience that I didn't anticipate after surgery.

"You need to get up and walk," the nursing staff cajoled me.

"I'm tired now. I'll do it later," I said barely audible to myself. My recovery was far more prolonged than I expected. Before surgery, I thought I'd be back to my old self in a matter of days. I was wrong.

"I'll be back in awhile," she said.

She was.

Since I already had taken a few trips around the hall with a physical therapist, I was deemed ready to go on my own. *I suppose it's better than looking at four white walls.* Being very active pre-surgery, I thought my energy would follow post-surgery. Wrong, again.

"I'm back," the nurse said cheerfully and with a smile. "How about you get up and walk around?"

I put on the robe that my son had brought me from home. Hospital gowns with their skimpy ties aren't exactly dignified. With slippers on, I started my walk alone.

There were noises and people in the hall, but I was scared. *What if I couldn't make it? What if I fell? Who would find me? What if? What if?*

So Walker and I took a stroll. As I rounded the corner, I saw out of the corner of my eye, a woman who had no visitors. She smiled at me. I carefully let go of one hand on the walker and waved.

"How are you?" she asked from her hospital bed.

"Good," I replied without conviction. Slowing my already unhurried pace, I hesitantly asked, "Do you want company?"

I know I did.

"Please come in," she said and pointed to the empty chair.

She was not allowed to go home until after she had heart surgery. Her problem was found during a routine angiogram. It didn't take long for me to hear the bitterness in her voice.

"So, where did you work?" she asked.

"I was a teacher for 38 years. Loved every minute of 37 of them. But I promised myself when I started teaching that the day I go to *work* instead of school is the day I think about retiring," I said staring at a spot on the wall that seemed to be playing a movie of my past life.

"I taught too," she said. "Where did you teach?"

"Niagara Wheatfield Schools, I was a reading teacher for kids in grades kindergarten to fifth grade. What about you?"

"Oh, I taught in Florida, North Carolina, Massachusetts," she said with a bit of agitation in her voice.

"Why so many places? I asked.

"It's where they sent me," she said with outright anger.

I didn't know whether I should ask, but I did.

"Who are they?" I questioned.

"The nuns, I was a nun," she said with a scowl on her face.

"I worked four years in a Catholic School in Buffalo," I said trying to form some connection. It didn't work. She was very sour on that time in her life.

We sat in silence, it wasn't uncomfortable because we both could hear the nurses' station and fellow cardiac patients walking the hall. When you're in a hospital, you get used to the quietness in your head.

"I got married, but he died. We were married for 30 years," she said.

I did what I do best. Listen and smile. I knew there was more and I was right.

"I have a boyfriend now."

I wondered how old this lady was. I didn't ask. I didn't have to.

"You'd think at my age, 83, I wouldn't have a boyfriend, but I do," she said with a quick smile that rapidly turned to a frown.

I wondered why the change in facial expression. I didn't have to wonder too long.

"Since I've been in this hospital, he has not called or come to see me." She paused and stared at the wall. "Not once," she said raising her finger with disgust.

"Well," I asked a bit unsure of whether I should ask. "Did you call him?"

"Yes," she said firmly, "and I'm not calling him again. He knows where I am."

More silence. More footsteps in the hall. I had unknowingly stirred up bad times for her. My walker was calling me and I was ready to take to the halls. She wasn't ready to let me go though.

"Do you have someone when you get home to help take care of you?" she questioned.

"Yes, I do," I didn't offer anymore. But she wanted more.

"Who?"

"My husband and my son. My son is coming in from New York City to help out."

"You're lucky. I have no one," she said tearfully.

"I'm sorry," I said.

I wanted to leave her with some comforting words. I'm not sure I believed them myself, but it didn't matter what I thought.

"Give him time. It's a lot to get used to. He'll call."

I slowly got up and made my way to my room.

Yeah, I was lucky. I had my family waiting for me. But I thought everyone did. I was mistaken. Up to that conversation, I never appreciated it either.

My Lesson Learned

People have all kinds of experiences in their suitcases. My luggage held both good and bad occurrences. I have people around me who care and I never appreciated it.

The Spirometer

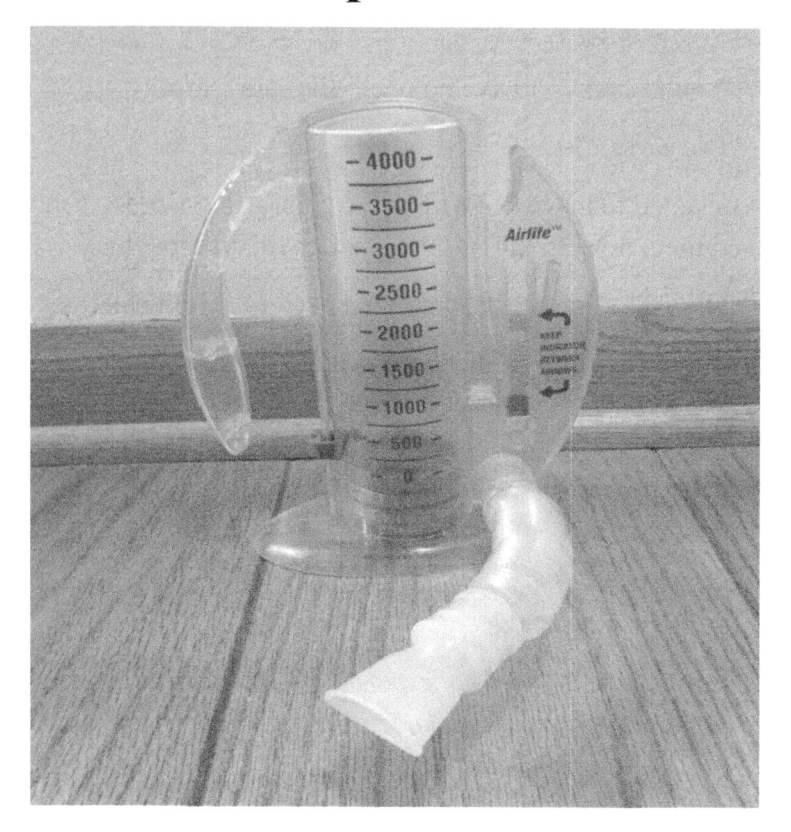

Photo courtesy of the author.

"Have you used your Spirometer today?" the nurse asked as she pumped my arm for another blood-pressure reading. I could hear the cuff expand as if each breath it took was on its own.

"Yes," I answered truthfully.

I grabbed the Spirometer, taking a deep inhale and watched the blue ball rise.

"How high did you get the ball?" she questioned as she removed the blood-pressure cuff from my arm.

Pointing to the spot, I said, "Right around here."

Placing her finger in a higher position, she said, "To avoid fluid in your lungs, you need to keep it at here,"

"Okay," I replied.

"I'm serious," she half scolded. "You don't want to have water in your lungs."

"Okay," I tried keeping the irritation out of my voice.

But I wasn't listening. It wasn't going to happen to me.

Until it did.

My Lesson Learned

Don't fake it. Do what the professionals ask even when you see no value in it.

Consequences

Having my lung tapped was very unpleasant. Could it have been avoided if I had used the Spirometer routinely? I knew if the doctor made a mistake, I'd have a bigger problem. Imagine someone sticking a long needle in your lung to remove water.

It is even difficult to write about the experience.

But I did ask to see what was pulled out of me. It looked like ½ quart of fluid.

Please, if you're reading this, do what the nurses tell you even when you might want to fake it.

My Lesson Learned

Blowing into a tube consistently may have saved me from having my lung tapped.

Leaving the Hospital

'Twas hours before leaving
And all through my mind
I thought of my own bed
Hoping fresh sheets I'd find.
When out in the hall,
I heard such a rattle.
A wheelchair arrived
With that I had battle.
I, in my determination
And they with their plan
Won the battle of the wheelchair
My stay ended like it began.
I sat in the wheelchair
Frustrated? You bet.
But I knew I was leaving
For home I was set.

Seven days later, an attendant wheeled me out the same door I entered, but with a repaired mitral valve.

Leaving the hospital had as many mandated procedures as getting admitted.

First mandate, I had a visit from the hospital pharmacist because I was temporarily put on Coumadin, a blood thinner. He explained the necessity of weekly blood draws to measure my INR (International Normalized Ratio). If my INR is too low, blood clots could form. If too high, there's an increased risk of bleeding. To combat this, my dose of Coumadin would vary depending on my food intake. Being asked to avoid green vegetables and salads is like asking a child to forgo ice cream. I nodded my head admitting that I understood. Being compliant is different from agreement, right?

Hydrocodone for pain was included in my go-home meds. I had every intention of not taking it, but to get out of the hospital I smiled and watched it placed in the go-home pile. When arriving home, it was safely disposed of.

Another pill, which met the same fate as Hydrocodone, was a pill that was given to me because according to their records I had gained too much weight. Another shake of the head. Actually I lost five pounds and I'm still angry that I paid for something that had the same destiny as the previous med.

With my foot-tapping its own beat, another knock on the door happened.

"Joanna?" she asked.

"Yes."

"I'm Beth, your discharge nurse. Can I go over a few things with you?"

Did she not see the pharmacist standing there? After a few seconds of awkward silence, the pharmacist spoke.

"We're done here. I just need you to sign this. It says I gave you all the meds you need and went over everything."

"Sure," I quickly glanced at the paperwork and did what I know is a no-no. I signed without reading. I wanted him out of the way. He shook my hand and left.

Beth moved in closer. I detected the scent of lemon coming from her uniform. Must be a common hospital procedure: I've smelled that pleasant odor before.

"Here are your discharge papers. I see the pharmacist talked to you so I'll check that off."

"Do you have any questions?"

"No," I had no idea what to ask.

"Let me go over everything," she said while adjusting the papers in her hand. "Here's a list of do's and don'ts. Take a minute to read through them."

The list included:

Don't carry anything more than five pounds for a month. (Grocery shopping?)

Don't go up and down stairs. (Laundry?)

Don't vacuum or do any heavy housework. (Dog hair?)

Be sure to watch your diet. You can't take a lot of Vitamin K.

She must have been watching my eyes read through as my next thought was What foods have Vitamin K? The next paper she slipped me listed foods high in Vitamin K. Kale, spinach, broccoli, Brussels sprouts, kiwi, and peas. All the foods I enjoy.

Her goal and my goal were different. I wanted out of the hospital and she wanted me to be an informed patient.

Next paper, the visiting nurse.

"I checked your insurance and you are eligible to have a nurse come and check your sutures and draw blood because you're on Coumadin. She'll answer any questions you may have."

I wonder if she can throw a load of laundry in while she's at it. Probably not.

"Last, no shower until the stitches are completely dissolved. The nurse will be checking for you."

"Okay," I replied. Asking her any questions meant a longer stay. I wanted my own home and bed.

"There's one last thing, if you notice any oozing from the area, contact your doctor immediately."

There are so many doctors involved; I had no idea who I would contact. I let that thought leave my head as quickly as it entered.

"How are you feeling now? Anything bothering you?"

At that moment, my husband walked in. "Ready?"

"Yes," I smiled.

"Sir," she said turning toward Paul. "Would you mind carrying her belongings to the car and I'll get Joanna ready to leave. By the time you get the car from the attendant, she'll be ready for you."

Paul grabbed my packed belongings and touched my shoulder before leaving.

"Now, let's look around and make sure you took everything. You'd be surprised at the number of people who leave cell phones, chargers and iPads," she said as she picked up magazines to make sure nothing was underneath.

"Looks good," she said.

As if on cue, an attendant pushing a wheelchair came into the room.

"We're just checking the room for her belongings," the nurse said to the attendant. "Everything looks good. Let me help you get in the wheelchair."

"I can do it. I don't need a wheelchair. I can walk."

"Hospital procedures," came the reply.

The elevator down from the 5th floor was quick. The attendant made small talk, but my mind traveled to the fresh air I would soon be smelling. Beyond the automatic glass door I spotted my husband sitting in the car.

"That's my husband," I said pointing.

"Okay, I'll just wheel you out," the attendant smiled.

"It's okay, I'll walk."

Expected reply, "Hospital procedures."

My Lesson Learned

Allowing hospital procedures to dictate my life was something I got use to. I knew it was happening and there was nothing I could do about it.

Visiting Nurse Appointment

The shrill sound from the phone startled me. I didn't recognize the number on the caller ID but did recognize the initials VNA. It was the Visiting Nurse Association. So I picked up. "Hello."

"Hi, my name is Cheryl and I'm calling from the VNA. Is Joanna there?"

I tried to hide my sleepy voice, foolishly embarrassed that I was not awake. "This is Joanna."

"How are you feeling today?" she asked.

"Fine. And you?"

"I'm good. Thank you. I'm calling to set up your first appointment with a visiting nurse. What days are good for you?"

For someone who feels confined in my own home, there are no bad days for visiting. I'm always here which is very different from my pre-surgery self. But before I answered her, my bank account voice kicked in, "What is the charge?"

"Let me check." I could hear the clicking coming from her computer. "Looks like zero co-pay."

I was skeptical. "For how long?"

More clicking came through the phone. "Until the nurse feels you are able to leave the house safely. You're not driving yet, are you?"

"No, not for at least six weeks," I said with a deep sigh.

"Then you'll have our services for at least six weeks. When can I set up the first appointment?"

Since my calendar was devoid of activities, I knew it didn't matter. But what did count is my early morning quiet time that I've had since a child. It was and is my time to become centered. To reflect on yesterday and to put right any wrongs today. I also listened for God's quiet voice. Sometimes it was so quiet, I didn't hear it.

"Any day after 10 A.M."

"How's tomorrow, Wednesday? We like to get to you as soon as possible when you are discharged from the hospital."

"Ok."

"You haven't taken a shower, have you?" she asked.

"No."

"Good, she'll let you know when you safely can." More clicking on the computer. "Looks like Amy has availability tomorrow morning. Amy will call before she comes and she will have ID on her." Cheryl said the phone number she had on file. "Is that correct?"

I thought to myself, "Well you called it and you're talking to me." But I kept my comments to myself and just said, "Yes." I was getting good at keeping my mouth shut.

"If you have any questions before tomorrow, call us. It was nice talking to you, Joanna."

With that we were disconnected. It always feels good to have someone call me by name instead of the 'patient in room 403.' I felt a smile flash across my face.

After hanging up, I asked myself when did it happen that I now require a visiting nurse? Wasn't it just yesterday when I played kickball with all the neighbor kids on my street? I can still hear the childhood accusations, "Quit stealing the base."

I sat down in my sunroom that faces my backyard. The birdfeeder was filled and my aviary friends came to visit. They went about their eating ritual as if I hadn't left for seven days. A mother robin gathering twigs for nest building reminded me of my home and the comfortable shell my parents provided. I can still feel my mother's hand on mine as she walked me down the street for my first day of kindergarten. Years later, she told me how she cried on the walk back home. As a parent, I can bring to mind my son's first day and how the bus driver didn't return him home. We panicked and called the school's bus garage. We saw a bus beeping and driving backwards down our street. The doors to the big yellow bus opened and out Jason came.

"What took you so long?"

"The bus driver asked where's the little guy that lives here." Jason said.

"Why didn't you get out?" Paul and I both asked.

"I'm not little, I'm big. Dad calls me big guy."

Didn't that just happen? How is it that he's now 32-years old? Time creeps up and before you know it, you have a visiting nurse.

My Lesson Learned

Each day that you are present is a present.

VNA Visit - Amy

Not able to take a shower bothered me. Although I gave myself a sponge bath, I felt dirty and disheveled. I put on clean pajamas. Being unsure as to what she needed to look at, I kept everything accessible.

Amy appeared promptly at 10 A.M. with a small-wheeled luggage and a computer. Her small stature didn't stop her from maneuvering her supplies. Since I'm unable to carry more than five pounds, I was forced to watch her struggle. Something I'm not used to.

"Sorry, I can't help you, but I can grab your computer," I offered.

"Thanks," Amy smiled as she handed me her laptop.

My dog, Sky, heard the commotion and as usual came up to her for a pat and a treat I had on the table.

"May I?" Amy asked pointing to the animal delight."

"Please do," I answered.

Sky gobbled it up and retreated to his spot in the back room. A fed dog is a happy dog.

"Can I get you a cup of tea or water?"

"No, thanks, let's get started."

She asked for all the insurance numbers, which I provided. Then she looked at the medications on the table. When my eyes fell on the pill bottles, I vowed to myself I would be off all of them as soon as safely possible. I like doing things naturally and these capsules were anything but.

"Let's take a look at your incision. May I?" she politely asked.

"Sure."

She smothered her hands with the liquid from a bottled hand sanitizer and snapped on blue surgical gloves.

I lifted my pajama top. Amy gently removed the white gauze covering my skin and delicately pressed on my right breast. When I looked down, I was shocked. My right breast was swollen and black and blue.. It was about a size D where my left breast was its normal B.

"Whoa, is that normal?" I questioned.

"Yes, the doctor went in through your right breast with his instrument. Being swollen and bruised is typical."

I added that to my 'I didn't know list.'

"What I'm doing now," she said as she continued to poke around, "is looking for any signs of infection."

My heart responded by its pounding. I crossed my legs and took a deep breath.

"Everything looks good." She swabbed my breast with alcohol and reapplied a dressing.

As I silently waited, she entered information on the computer. Looking at me, she said, "Because you are on Coumadin, I need to check your INR levels, okay?"

"Yes," I said but had no idea how that would be done.

She fiddled in her luggage and came up with a syringe. The confused look on my face spoke to her.

"Oh, you didn't know how I would do the testing?"

"No," I answered.

"I'm going to clean the area," she said pointing to my right arm by the elbow, "and draw some blood."

She looked at me. I nodded to let her know I understood.

"Then I'll drop it off at Quest and I'll call your doctor for the results tomorrow morning."

"That fast?" I questioned.

"You have to be careful when you're on Coumadin. You want just the right amount. Not too much, not too little. If there's a problem, your doctor will call you."

"What does INR mean?"

"It stands for International Normalized Ratio," she said.

"And what does that mean?" I thought back to my teaching days and all the terms we used sometimes without explanation in front of parents.

"Well, 1.1 or below is normal range. If your numbers are higher, then your blood clots slower than we'd want. If your numbers are lower, your blood clots more quickly than we'd want."

"Does that have something to do with Vitamin K?" I asked.

"Yes, it does. Vitamin K normally helps your blood clot. Coumadin works against Vitamin K making your blood clot more slowly. If you eat a lot of salads, we have to be careful."

I didn't say it, but I'm a salad a day person. I also remember being told be cautious when eating salads. I didn't listen. There were so many restrictions and I wanted my salad.

She went to my right arm. At least I didn't have to argue with her about using my left arm. Before I knew it, my blood was drawn and she attached pre-made labels that were in a folder labeled with my name.

"Can we look at calendars and schedule our next visit?" Amy asked.

Getting up, I got my wall calendar, devoid of any activity, hanging in my bedroom.

"Anything after 10 A.M.," I said adhering to keeping my personal meditation time sacred.

"In the beginning, I'll see you 3-times a week. The phlebotomist will set up an appointment to draw blood," she added.

"You just drew it. Why can't you?"

"I can. But that's her job."

"I understand. But it's easier for me to schedule one visit," I said knowing I had nowhere to go.

Part of me felt badly as I knew I was cutting into someone's paid hours. But I didn't want different people coming in and out of the house.

"I suppose I could," Amy relented.

"Thank you."

We scheduled two weeks' worth of visits. Before packing up, she said, "Do you have any questions for me?"

"Not a question. But I am very tired most of the time."

"Joanna, you had major surgery and your body is trying to repair itself. It does that while at rest."

"When will I feel like myself again?" I pushed a fallen hair from my face.

"Couple months, at least a couple of months."

I didn't like the answer. I thought I would get off the operating table and resume my normal life.

Amy zipped up the vials of blood and placed them in her luggage. She checked her cell phone that had been on silent.

"I'll be back in two days. Don't be afraid to rest. You've earned it."

I heard her car start, then she drove away to her next appointment. My decision was to follow her advice. I fell asleep.

Before dozing off, I thought about Amy. She was consistent and punctual for the entire six weeks. I found myself looking forward to her visits even though I knew she would poke me for a blood test.

There's something to be said about human contact when you're ill. As a healthy person, I never thought about my friendships. I believed they'd always be there. For the most part, people were by my side. Even people I didn't expect to hear from sent a card or a gift. I knew Amy would be a transient friend, but she always came with a smile and left me happily grinning when she left.

There was a knock on my door during one of Amy's visits. A flower shop owner had a bouquet of flowers for me from a friend. Something else to make the day brighter.

During my convalescence, I received many get-well gifts that to this day, I treasure the thoughtfulness. I tucked it away on my necessary 'to do' list. When a friend is sick, I need to remember to do something kind for that person.

Amy was one of the gifts I received weekly. I wanted the six weeks to end so I could drive, but I didn't want to terminate the friendship. But it was time for me to go it alone.

My checkups happened outside of my protected shell. I felt like a turtle, sticking my head out a little bit at a time to check my surroundings. Time to do more waiting in a 'waiting room.' My period of being taken care of was ending. It was time to take care of myself.

My Lesson Learned

Sometimes your body demands rest. I needed to shut up, quit arguing with myself and obey.

Pre-Cardiac Rehab

After my visiting nurse was no longer visiting, it was time to get a recheck by Dr. Heart. When I called for an appointment, I was able to get in quickly.

Paul and I went together again for this meeting. Same routine, sign up, hand over co-pay, take a seat, and then hope you'll be called close to your time. I'm usually in sooner rather than later.

Dr. Heart suggested cardiac rehab as part of a protocol for getting myself back in shape again.

"You don't have to do this, Joanna, but patients that do, are on the mend quicker," Dr. Heart said.

"Where do I go?" I asked.

Handing me a slip of paper, I saw listings for places next to my house.

"Anyone of these is good. It's personal preference. Now let me listen to your heart."

Using the stethoscope, he placed the diaphragm on my heart and asked me to breathe and hold. I was getting used to this procedure. He then placed the chest piece on my back with the same directions.

"Breathe and hold please," came the instructions. "Everything sounds good. How are you feeling?" he asked with genuine concern.

"Tired most of the time."

"That's very normal. You had major surgery. If you decide to go to cardiac rehab, you'll begin to gain your strength back."

Paul, who had been quiet, spoke, "I think it's a good idea. It'll get you out of the house and get you stronger."

Dr. Heart chimed in, "Would you like a script for it?"

My hesitation lasted a few seconds. "Yes."

"Your heart sounds good, Joanna. Come and see me in another six months. Always feel free to come sooner if you have any questions."

He shook our hands before leaving and said, "It was nice seeing both of you again."

Paul and I left the office and before driving away, we both agreed. "What a nice guy he is."

My Lesson Learned

There are still genuine caring doctors in the profession of cardiac care. My doctor looks at me and not at a computer screen. I am lucky to have him.

Sometimes Family is Right

It was time to visit after convalescing for a couple of weeks.

Outfitted in my pajamas and a summer robe complete with bedroom slippers, I waited for my sister to drive me to my niece's house 15 minutes away. Unusual clothes? Yes. I wanted to be comfortable and it was one of my first trips out of the house.

"What are you wearing? Why aren't you dressed?" my sister Maria asked.

"I am dressed. I'm comfortably dressed," I answered.

She shook her head and shrugged her shoulders. I fastened my seat belt. Away we went.

I wanted to see a different environment. I needed to see people whom I would feel relaxed with. So, I became comfy in my clothes, that's how I wanted to feel with my family.

Although I had taken these roads many times, this felt different. I noticed things I hadn't seen before

As we pulled into the driveway, I noticed my niece's landscaping. Pretty flowers, and bushes lined the front of her house. The porch swing swaying back and forth reminded me of how free I use to feel.

I rang the doorbell and I heard footsteps padding across her floor.

"Well, look who's here?" my niece, Shannon, said. Then she followed it with, "WHAT do you have on?"

"I want to be comfortable," I answered.

"Well, you do look comfy," she replied.

I found my way to the couch, sat, and looked around. Nothing had changed, except for me. The photos on the walls took on new meaning. I looked at everything differently. I felt like I came back from the dead. In a way, I did, since my heart was stopped during surgery in order to repair my mitral valve. That still freaks me out to think of it.

The hours passed with chitchat. Talk of what to have for lunch happened.

Shannon said, "I'm going to go to the store. What do you need Josie?" she used my nickname that my family gave me.

"Nothing really, but I'll come too."

"Like that?" my sister and niece spoke in unison.

"Yeah, why not?"

"If you go out like that, people are going to think you escaped from a home and the cops will be called," my sister said.

Shannon nodded in agreement.

"They will not. I'm fine. So what if I have pajamas on?" I said with a bit of attitude.

"I'm NOT taking you," my niece said. "I'll buy you what you need, but you're not coming with me dressed like that."

That was settled, I wasn't going anywhere. Now as I look back on that day, I realize I wasn't thinking clearly. I'm grateful that they were.

What made me think it was okay to go out dressed in my pajamas complete with bedroom slippers? When my heart was repaired, did they do something to my rational thought process? Were the medications I consumed causing me to lose common sense? I'm not sure. But I do know, I'm glad they didn't let me go shopping in my sleeping attire.

My Lesson Learned

Although I was miffed at the time, I'm thankful they stuck to their convictions and I wasn't allowed out of the house dressed in pajamas. I'm glad my family made the right decision when I couldn't.

Embarrassed

I'm ashamed of what I'm about to write, but it's the truth. Shopping at any store, I'd notice people who looked healthy in motorized scooters. I wondered why are you on that thing? Walk, it's better for you, my self-righteous voice spoke.

I don't consider myself a judgmental person. Actually I think I'm pretty kind. But don't all critical people think they're caring?

It was about six weeks after my mitral valve surgery and I was given the okay to drive. Time to put on my big girl pants. I lost confidence doing the very simple things, like driving a car. But I decided I needed some things at a store, so I drove myself.

I parked as close as I could to the entrance of the store, which is something I rarely did pre-surgery. Walking is good, I'd tell myself. Not today, I cruised around for a close parking spot. I sped up if I thought the person coming toward me wanted the space that I hunted for. When the doc fixed my heart, did he change it in anyway, I wondered. Someone else had residence in my body. I didn't recognize her.

The aisles seemed longer than I remembered. People moved slowly and they were in my way. I wanted to get in and get out. My patience left me and I didn't know how to find it.

After shopping, which lasted not longer than ten minutes, I was wiped out. Not sweating droplets, but physically exhausted. I couldn't carry much, only the five pounds that was medically allotted to me so my shopping bag was light.

I looked healthy, no cane, no limping, no outward sign of a problem. But I was struggling. Anyone looking at me would not know that I was having a hard time. Walking out of the store, I realized I might not make it to my car. Then I spotted a 'lifesaver', a motorized scooter. All plugged in and ready to move. I left the electricity connected, but knew I needed a rest. With my meager bag by my side, I sat in the scooter. Getting quick glances my way from passersby, I ignored the stares. I realized I might have done the same thing pre-surgery. What is this healthy woman doing taking up a scooter for a person who needs it?

I noticed many able-bodied people and wondered if they appreciated their health. I know I didn't when I was healthy. As I sat on the scooter with my meager bag by my side, passersby gave me disapproving glances. I ignored their stares. Mothers dragging children with one hand and dads grabbing the hand of another child. Their whole life in front of them. Up until now, I was like them. Not anymore.

Now, I'm limited and sitting in a motorized scooter that is getting powered up for the next person in need.

After a few minutes, I meandered to my car. Fortunately I remembered where I parked it. I didn't have to go too far. I was never so glad to see it.

My Lesson Learned

People in scooters are there for a reason. Grab the can of tomatoes they're struggling to get while seated. Someone may need to grab one for me some day.

Cardiac Rehab

Having little to no sense of direction even with a GPS that often recalculates, I chose a hospital, since I knew exactly where I would be going. And I also figured what better place to be if things go south in a hurry. Just wheel me over.

Cardiac rehab was located on the 3rd floor. You can't use the stairs. Another hospital regulation. I hate elevators. Having a phobia about being locked in a tall rising metal box with strangers is where I'm at. But after exiting my car and locating the box, I walked into the hoist, pressed the three and watched and heard the steel against steel. I don't know what's worse; being alone or sharing space with a stranger. My eyes gazed at the numbers, two, and then three. Sudden thump and then relief when the steel door opened. I noticed a sign pointing to cardiac rehab and there was a receptionist's desk. No line, she looked up, smiled and said, "How may I help you?"

"I'm here for cardiac rehab," I said.

"Name?" she asked.

"Joanna Torreano."

Her finger slid across a paper and stopped at my name.

"There you are. Welcome Joanna."

"Thanks," although I didn't feel thankful.

After taking my insurance information and co-pay, she took me to a room with a table and chairs. There was one vacant seat. All of the people surrounding the table looked older than I. It reaffirmed my questioning mind as to what was I doing here. The people seemed to know each other inquiring about each other's families. A man turned to me, extended his hand, "Marc," he said.

"Joanna," I replied.

"First time?" he questioned.

"Yeah."

"It's a bit intimidating. This is a nice group of people. You'll be okay."

Was my nervousness that obvious? Looking around the room, I saw cards of appreciation on the walls. A picture of a heart with labeled parts shared the same surface. At exactly 10 A.M., a pleasant nurse came in and gave us one of several lectures we'd have on the heart. These lectures were held on the first Monday of the month. After the lesson, blood pressure and heart rate were taken and noted on a chart that I would carry around with me.

Before exercising, I had to wear a heart monitor. Adorning the wall was a picture with colored leads so I would know where to place them. After placing them, I had to sit quietly to get a normal baseline. Not sure how ordinary it was since I felt like a caged animal with other creatures sharing my space.

Every person had an individual program: five different machines with eight-minute intervals. Piece of cake, *I'm in good shape*. Wrong again, I 'had been' in good shape. I needed to get back in shape.

Next stop, workout room. Each machine had buttons that controlled the degree of resistance and in some instances the rate at which the equipment would operate.

My first step was the treadmill. The nurse punched in the speed and resistance. It was much lower than my pre-surgery self. But I kept my thoughts to myself. I was getting good at that.

Inserting the earbuds from my iPhone into my ears I wanted to escape. My desertion lasted seconds.

"Excuse me," the nurse said. "We don't allow any distractions. Hospital regulations. Please remove the earbuds," she said smiling.

Why it made a difference, I don't know. But I removed the 'disruption' and watched the time tick down from the eight minutes.

At one point during each session, my blood pressure was taken while I used an exercise machine. The numbers were noted on the chart I walked around with.

When I was done with the machines, my next step was the hall. I had to make two rounds of the area while I was monitored. I'm not sure if the nurse was there to check on my compliance or to make sure I didn't fall over. But I felt like cattle going around the ring.

There were hand sanitizer containers placed on the walls for convenience. I didn't use them. I prefer soap and water. Probably another mandated procedure that I could finally choose to ignore.

Final stop is where I began. I sat around the table and had my blood pressure and heart rate taken again. Did I return to normal, whatever that is.

Cardiac rehab continued for several months. It did get easier, but my fear of elevators never went away. Something caused my fear of elevators to subside. I didn't have to use the elevator. I got kicked out of cardiac rehab.

My Lesson Learned

Getting out of my comfort zone was uncomfortable. But to gain physical strength, I had to gain mental stamina.

Cardiac Flunkie

I got kicked out of cardiac rehab. Have you ever heard of such a thing? No, I didn't misuse a machine. I had high blood pressure.

"Joanna," the nurse said. "I'm going to send you home today," she said as she pulled the Velcro cuff from my arm.

"Why?" I had the 'guilty' syndrome while being innocent.

"Your blood pressure is too high. I don't want you exercising."

"Then what?" I asked. "How do I get it down?"

"You'll have to make an appointment with your primary or cardiac doctor to figure it out," she offered.

During this conversation, the other cardiac patients busied themselves by staring at their fingernails.

"I'm sorry, but hospital regulations. I could get in trouble if I let you stay," she said with compassion.

She must have read my mind because her next words were, "You'll get a credit for the co-pay today."

I took my car keys from the table, barely smiled at my fellow cardiac patients and said, "Well, good-bye everyone."

Their nail staring ended and in unison said, "Good-bye Joanna."

Elevator time again. This time, I wasn't sure if I'd ever have to use it again. I felt dejected and scared. If I can't exercise to get better, how would I regain my strength?

Unlocking my car door, I slid in the front seat with hunched shoulders and thought, "Now what?"

Pulling into the driveway, Paul was just about in his car ready to head out, "You're home early," he said.

"Yeah, well, I was kicked out," I said.

"No, really, why are you home?" he asked.

"Not kidding. My blood pressure is too high and I was told 'hospital regulations,' I can't exercise."

"So what are you supposed to do?" he asked as he leaned against his car.

"I guess I have to call either Dr. Primary or Dr. Heart."

"Come on, let's go in the house and figure this out." Paul said.

"But you're on your way out?"

"It's okay. Come on."

We ambled in together.

My Lesson Learned

Two heads are better than one-especially when one is in the medical profession.

High Blood Pressure

Paul and I talked it through and I called my primary doctor since she's easier to get into and a closer drive. Dialing the number, and after a few rings, I heard, "Doctor's office, how may I help you?"

I explained my situation. "How's today at 3:30?" she asked.

"Perfect."

Since it was 11:30, I didn't have that long to fret and worry.

"She'll probably put you on a high blood pressure med," Paul offered.

"I don't want it," I said.

"You also don't need the complications from not taking anything such as…"

I cut him off. "Okay, okay, point made."

As in all marriages, sometimes it's good to walk away. Grabbing his keys, he said, "I'll be back at 4 or so, and we can take the dog for a walk."

"Okay," I said.

I did not Google high blood pressure or medications. Living with someone who knew the medical consequences was enough for me.

Driving to the appointment, I felt discouraged. I knew I felt fine, more than fine. My heart that use to reverberate through me is as quiet as leaves falling. *What is going on that I'm not aware of?*

Shutting off my car and grabbing my purse, I made my way to the glass window that separates me from the receptionist. I gave her my name and insurance information. She pointed to the right, "Have a seat, Doctor will be with you shortly."

My doctor is good and punctual. Within minutes, I heard, "Joanna?"

As I followed the nurse in, she pointed to the scale. Same routine. Then directed me to a room.

"So what brings you here?" she asked.

I filled her in and she entered my responses into the computer.

"Let's take your blood pressure now." She placed the cuff on my arm and pumped air into it. After a few seconds, I heard the air wheeze out.

"140 over 90," she said with a routine voice.

"Is that high?" I asked.

"Doctor will go over it with you," she politely, but non-committedly answered. "Any other questions?"

"No," I thought why ask when I wouldn't be given answers.

She left and I stared at the framed child's drawing on the wall. Nice touch. Slight knock on the door and Dr. Primary came in and warmly shook my hand.

"Nice to see you, Joanna," she said. "I read the notes so I know why you are here. Let me take a listen for myself." She placed the cuff on my arm and my results were higher.

"White coat syndrome," I said and then added, "Minus the white coat."

She always wore street clothes.

"I'd like to recommend Lisinopril, it's a high blood pressure medication. But to make sure I'm not missing anything, I'd like you to see Dr. Heart."

Another 50 bucks I thought. But I told myself to shut up.

"High blood pressure is typical after surgery. Don't worry. I like to be careful."

Her thoroughness has kept me from a life without oxygen.

"Same pharmacy?" she asked.

"Yes."

"I'll send it over right now. Give them some time to fill it. And Joanna, don't worry." Another handshake and she left.

I headed out to a local coffee shop and continued writing this book.

My Lesson Learned

Curve balls happen in life. It's hard when it's unexpected. But I guess that's why it's called a curve.

Dr. Heart - High Blood Pressure

I gave myself a day to relax and not make any phone calls.

After a few days, Paul nonchalantly asked, "So have you called Dr. Heart?"

"Doing it today," I said.

He touched my shoulder and walked away. Here we go again. I dialed the number and a receptionist answered and asked me the purpose of my call. I filled her in. "I have an opening tomorrow at 4:30. It's his last appointment of the day."

"Okay," I said.

I wanted to go alone. I don't know why. But I did.

Hating thruways, I went the long way. Reaching the door, it felt heavier than usual. Probably my demeanor, I decided. Handing over 50 bucks again for another look at me was frustrating. The wait for the visit was minimal.

"Joanna," I heard.

Another step on the scale and she pointed to the room on the left.

"So what brings you here?" she asked.

As I talked, she put notes into the computer. She prepared me for an EKG. Not sure if she read any notes, but she mentioned her son who is struggling in reading.

"Tell me about your son. How is he struggling?" I asked.

"Reading, he doesn't comprehend."

Right up my alley. I might be a retired reading teacher, but my concern and knowledge were still intact. I gave her suggestions.

"I'm very interested in what you have to say, but you must remain still for a few seconds while I do this EKG."

After a few seconds, the testing was complete. Removing the adhesive leads, we continued chatting. It felt good to use my wisdom to help someone.

"Thank you, you've been very helpful," she said as she backed the EKG machine out of the room. "Dr. Heart will be right with you."

It felt good to disengage from the present. I heard a slight tap on the door and reality again.

"Joanna," Dr. Heart extended his hand.

"Back again," I said with a little punch.

"I've read the notes and your EKG came back normal. Now, let me listen to your heart."

Earpiece in, chest-piece on my heart and I did the usual with his instructions.

"Take a deep breath, hold, and slowly exhale."

I could write the manual. I knew exactly what to do.

"Everything sounds good. So, you were kicked out of cardiac rehab?"

"Yeah," I said feeling like I did something wrong to deserve it.

"I see that your primary put you on Lisinopril," he said as a statement.

"I hate taking that stuff," I said.

"It could only be temporary. Keep taking it and you may be able to wean yourself off. What you're going through is normal, Joanna. Your heart sounds good, your EKG came back fine. You had major surgery and the body takes some time to repair itself."

"Why is it acting up now? I've been in rehab for a while."

"That I don't know. But I do know, you'll get through this and your heart is in good shape."

Ever the cheerleader, I like this guy.

"If you don't have any further questions, I'll have your primary follow this. I'll send over a report so she'll know nothing is wrong with your heart. I'll send a copy to cardiac rehab clearing you to go back," he paused for a second. "Please come in if you have any further concerns. I'm here."

"Thanks," and I extended my hand.

We shook and he backed out of the door.

My Lesson Learned

Sometimes 50 bucks is worth the price for peace of mind. I had to accept the fact that for a while I have to take a med.

Return to Cardiac Rehab

Being cleared by the cardiologist to return to cardiac rehab, I dialed the number to see if there were any available slots.

"Cardiac rehab, Libby speaking, how may I help you?" she said.

"This is Joanna Torreano and I was… um… kicked out of rehab,… umm….due to high blood pressure," I stammered through.

She was not fazed. "Date of birth?" she asked.

I gave her the information.

"Oh, there you are. I see you have a credit on your account."

That was music to my ears. I heard papers shuffling. "Let's see what we have," tapping pencil sounds came through the phone. "Looks like the Monday, Wednesday, Friday slots are available. How's that?"

"When would I start?" I asked.

"You can start tomorrow if you'd like. Can I put you in?"

"Sure. Thanks."

"See you tomorrow at 10. You don't need to go through registration since I have all of your information."

I heard the phone click and I felt relief and panic. What if I get kicked out again? My head was filled with self-imposed uneasiness.

Restless sleep was next. I felt like a child who misbehaved and was now allowed back on the swing set. I didn't want to be pushed too hard, but wanted just enough momentum to get me moving.

The dreaded elevator was another hurdle I had to re-encounter.. When the doors opened, I intentionally walked slower than usual to the workout room hoping to lower my blood pressure. I became good at playing mind games with my heart.

Opening the door, I saw familiar faces mixed with a few unexpected patients.

"Hey, you're back," a few people said.

"Yeah," I said hoping the nurse had seen my clearance to attend.

'Be good,' I silently told my heart.

Blood pressure cuff on, air pumped in, released and numbers were written on my chart.

She was on to the next patient.

I made it.

Entering the workout room, I felt like I had never left. My first assignment was the treadmill. This time I did not wear my earbuds. I did not grab a magazine like I wanted. I learned to follow the rules I didn't know existed. Looking around the room, I saw all the other patients working on various machines, as if I had never left. The nurse went from patient to patient measuring blood pressure during the workout. I was concerned when she got to me. Would my blood pressure be too high? Would I be sent home again? Just thinking those thoughts may cause my blood pressure to rise.

Calm down, Joanna. Calm down.

The resistance and incline on the treadmill were lower than when I left. It was my turn. Blood pressure cuff on, air pumped in, and a slow release. She wrote down numbers, smiled, gave me a thumbs up and went on to the next person.

Two times today, I made the cut.

After our five-machine workout, we had to walk the hall. Up and back, up and back. I opted out of using the disinfectant pump after using the machines, preferring good old-fashioned water and soap. Then back to the original room where blood pressure was taken again. I never realized how many times I was being monitored not including the heart monitor I wore for rehab.

Here we go again. She came to me last. Maybe hoping to make sure I was rested. Same procedure. Cuff on, air pressure in cuff, and a slow release. I felt the air escape and some from my mouth too as I unconsciously held my breath.

Another thumbs up.

Three for three. I could return next week. Time to meet the elevator again.

My Lesson Learned

Since the 'What ifs' never happened, I wonder how less stressful my life would be if I didn't entertain "What ifs?"

Last Day of Cardio Rehab

Phase III

The crunch of the hard snow under my feet seemed louder than usual. The frigid temperatures reached my ears and fingers quicker than I had remembered in the past. The automatic door wasn't frozen and I got a blast of warm air as I entered the hospital's cardiac center. I stomped my feet on the carpeting to remove as much snow as I could. I think I woke the receptionist.

Having wet feet, I walked gingerly on the tiled floor hoping I'd stay upright. I made it. *Who needs a broken hip?*

Pressing the button for the third floor on the elevator reminded me of how much I hate that metal box. Just one more day. Up, up, it went and after a slight pause, the door opened. I let out a deep breath I didn't know I was holding. I heard the sound of voices before I entered the room. I took in all the friendly faces knowing that today was my last day. Six men and two women were ready for the 40 minute workout that began and ended with blood pressure and heart rate monitoring as the first and last step.

Music from the 70s and 80s playing in the background from the CD player kept me company. I don't usually do this, but today I sang along. Some people around me were chatting and others were in their own thoughts. I was amusing myself by singing along pretty much in tune.

As I went from machine to machine, I thought back to my first day at cardiac rehab where eight minutes per machine seemed difficult.

Today, I did my workout effortlessly, which made me realize I should probably push myself harder.

"Why are you leaving? Don't you like us?" was asked over and over.

"No, it's not that. I belong to two gyms and I exercise regularly," I paused. "It's just time," I said with a deep sigh.

"Oh, I thought you didn't like us," came the two-person response.

I did like them, but being there reminded me of my reason for joining. I was feeling better and needed to remove myself from the memory of April 24th, my surgery date. Feeling confident that my blood pressure was stable and my heart rate was within range, I knew it was time for me to go it alone.

Each machine I completed brought me closer to the finish line. Or was it a beginning line? I'd be on my own to accomplish what I had started at cardiac rehab. I looked around at the familiar faces and hugged my new friends good-bye.

I walked slower to the elevator and took in all the sights and sounds. I saw people lingering for stress tests. People waiting to use the machines I just left behind. I pushed the button on the elevator to go down. As I slowly descended, I was pleased when the elevator door opened. I stepped out and heard the slamming of the metal door behind me.

The automatic door noticed me and the frigid air blasted me back into my new reality. I got in my car, turned the key, and drove away feeling bittersweet. Would I remain as dedicated to my own health as I did when I was paying for it? Only time would tell.

My Lesson Learned

Greet each new experience as just that, a new experience. It's true, when one door shuts, look for another to open. I'm okay with that, as long as it's not an elevator door.

Post-Stress Test

I had to go back in the elevator. This time, not for cardiac rehab, but for a post-stress test. Once again, I sat in the 'waiting' room. After 35 minutes, I was aggravated, but ready.

What happened to being on time especially when dealing with testing of the heart? Doesn't aggravation equal distress? I was at the hospital early for my 11 o'clock appointment. I heard laughter coming from the break room. Then I saw the door being closed. Before it shut, happy voices filtered their way to me. But my exasperation blocked them.

Then a nurse approached me, "Okay, Joanna, we're ready for you," said the smiling nurse.

We walked just a few feet into the room. "Please put your stuff down," she said pointing to a table. "Then sit up on the bed," she said as she spread fresh sheets on. "I have to ask you a few questions and then we'll get started."

The requests were routine. Name, date of birth, and any allergies. She was trying to make me feel comfortable and I decided to let go of my irritation and let her.

"Okay, now let me explain what's going to happen. You've had a stress test before, right?"

"Yes."

"Well, when we're done, I'm going to be able to tell you what your target heart rate should be." I'm going to clean the area first where I'll be putting on the leads. Would you mind laying down?"

I did as asked. She was very professional and made small talk. She took a tube and put the ingredients on a cotton swab and cleaned up the area where the leads were going. "Almost done."

She placed the leads on my chest and paged the doctor who must be there while I was being tested. He brought a student with him.

"Okay, we're ready. What's going to happen is you will be on the treadmill and in two minute intervals, it's going to get harder." She put the grade up to ten.

"Ten?" I asked, "Already?"

"Don't worry, we're going to be monitoring you. If it's too hard, we'll back it off."

The doctor moved closer to the machine that was producing squiggly lines. I had no idea what he was looking at. But I asked.

"How am I doing? Am I passing?"

"Fine, fine," the Asian doctor said smiling.

Before I knew it, I was up to a grade of 12. "Are you trying to kill me?" I asked to lighten up the mood.

I got the expected laughter. "Hey, I'm still talking and walking. I guess I'm doing okay."

But then I wasn't. "Okay," I said turning to the nurse and doctor. "I think I've had enough."

"A few more minutes," was the quick reply.

I didn't think I could handle anymore. I imagined myself fainting or falling or doing both.

Suddenly the treadmill slowed down. I took a deep breath and felt relieved that I was done.

"Well, did I pass?" I asked to no one in particular.

"Yes," was the two-person reply.

Results were given immediately and I learned that after attending cardiac rehab for 36 sessions, I had improved.

But most important to me was I felt like I was a person. I was congratulated on my progress and left feeling better than when I walked through the door.

My Lesson Learned

There is kindness in the medical profession. I had to be open to it. Cardiac Rehab was worth the time and money. Without it, recuperation would have been longer.

Cardio without Monitoring

Although I'm disciplined, I missed my cardio-friends. I decided to pay monthly for cardio without monitoring. My blood pressure would be taken before working out, but nothing during or after. I guess it's a weaning process.

Even though I didn't know much about my exercise mates personally, our common bond of heart issues held us together.

Some had stints, others had had heart attacks. My surgery seemed to be minor compared to others. I also got the 'newer' award being 10-20 years younger than my exercise mates.

I noticed the cards lining the walls from previous patients. Some were in 'memory' of which caused me to pause.

It hit me how I used this block of time as a wall around myself. I didn't have to go out and meet new people. We shared a commonality. But reality set in. With people coming and going, there was no opportunity to form lasting friendships. Once they left, that was it.

Seeing someone at a local park made me stop and think. *Where do I know this guy from?* He must have noticed the quizzical look on my face. Pointing to his heart, he said, "Cardiac Rehab." We exchanged pleasantries asking each other how we were doing. But then we moved on.

I stayed only a month with cardio without monitoring. It was time to nurture other relationships.

My Lesson Learned

Being comfortable isn't always healthy.

Eye Appointment for Black Dot

My heart was beating like a rapid drum. I tried to portray a person in charge, but I was failing.

Before walking in the eye doctor's office, I had called my primary and heart doctor only to be told, "This is an issue for your eye doctor."

That was something I learned over and over. There were too many people involved in my care and the problem (me) was shifted from person to person. Ever since having mitral valve repair surgery, I have been experiencing different eye issues. The latest was a black spot about the size of a dime that floated in my right eye. My vision was temporarily affected for about five seconds. I was tired of going from doctor to doctor so I figured I just let this go. But my husband had other thoughts.

"You can't do nothing. You need to find out why this is happening," my husband Paul said with resolve in his voice.

"I'm okay, it's nothing," I replied.

"You don't know that. Just go in and find out," he said with what felt like a stronger opinion. With that, he grabbed his car keys to go out for the day.

The problem? Who was going to see me? I started with my primary and was told someone would get back to me. My phone rang. My primary suggested I see the cardiologist. The cardiologist had other ideas. He suggested the eye doctor. I looked up his phone number and called.

"Doctor's Office, can I help you?"

"This is Joanna Torreano and I'm having a black dot that temporarily obscures my vision. Is it possible to get in today?"

"Let me check. He's busy 'til the end of our office hours. But I know he'd want to see you. Can you come in at 5?"

"Sure, no problem."

I hung up, but the deafening sound of the phone ringing occurred again. This time it was the receptionist for the eye doctor.

"Doctor would like you to come in at 2 o'clock incase he needs to refer you, can you do that?"

I hesitated for only a second since I didn't know where his new office was and I have no sense of direction.

"Sure, " I said with more enthusiasm than I felt.

I quickly went out to my car and started my Garmin. Nothing, dead. The temperature read 2 degrees. Battery must be frozen. I remembered I had my phone with Google Maps. Easy solution, but I didn't know how to use Google Maps. So I used Mapquest and figured out how to get from my house to the doctor's office.

My mind was racing. Why did he want to see me so soon? If he referred me, how was I to get to the office? Having no sense of direction has been very frustrating for all of my life. Thruway driving, forget it. I'll take side roads.

I was nervous and going alone since my husband rarely turned on his seldom-used cell phone.

Armed with written directions and a strong sense of purpose, I was happy that I didn't have to take the thruway. Before leaving the house, I memorized the way, right, left, left. I arrived at 1:45, fifteen minutes ahead of schedule. I opened the office door and was greeted with a warm smile. "Your directions were perfect," I said returning the kind smile. I sat down and the office door opened. It was the doctor.

"Hi Joanna, I'll be with you in a minute." Within minutes, I was sitting in the chair.

"What seems to be the problem?" he asked.

"My eyes have not been the same since my surgery, April 24th. Recently a black spot, the size of a dime has been affecting my vision for a few seconds."

"Let's take a look," he said as he placed stinging drops in both of my eyes.

"Place your chin on here," he said pointing to a white plastic holder.

After giving me a thorough exam, he told me he wanted my eyes dilated more.

"Can you sit in the waiting room for 15 minutes and then I'll take another look?" he asked.

"Sure."

I went to my car to get sunglasses.

Fifteen minutes is not a long time unless you're waiting for health news. Then each minute seems to be longer. I was called in for my second exam and the doctor announced, "I'm very certain that your eyes are fine. I don't know why you are having these symptoms," he paused. "Maybe you should see your cardiologist."

"He told me to see you," I quickly replied. "I feel like a ping pong ball that keeps getting swatted, and is in the air and never lands."

There was a brief silence. "If it happens again, let him know that your eyes exam showed healthy eyes," he waited and appeared to be measuring his words. "Perhaps your mitral valve is acting up."

I left with mixed emotions. I had healthy eyes, but the problem remained. I put my sunglasses on to help with the glare.

I had to reverse the directions I had memorized to get to the doctor. I pulled into my driveway wondering when the symptoms would reoccur.

The black dots never came back. I have no idea why, but decided it was time to let that worry go.

My Lesson Learned

Follow through on everything even if it feels pointless. Peace of mind is its own reward.

Linda

After six weeks of recovery, I received a phone call from my dear friend, Linda.

"How about if you come over for lunch?" she asked. "I'll invite Lisa too."

"Sure," I said without hesitation. I was ready to see someone other than doctors or nurses. No poking for blood, no cold stethoscope on my repaired heart.

With permission to drive and able to turn the steering wheel, I felt some trepidation. My confidence had taken a hit. I was afraid of car horns, traffic lights and a possible finger from an irritated motorist.

Arriving safely without being recalculated by my GPS, I parked in Linda's driveway. Getting out of my car, I took a moment to savor the wind blowing past me. An insistent red cardinal didn't stop squawking until my eyes met his. For me, a red cardinal signals a visit from someone who passed away. Who was visiting me? The smell of something Italian hit my nose as I walked to Linda's screened door. Seeing no doorbell, I gently knocked. Hearing footsteps coming my way, Linda greeted me with, "So, you found my new home?"

My lack of directions is universally known with my friends. She opened the door and the Italian scent fully filled my nostrils and my stomach quickly responded with a loud growl.

"Sounds like someone is hungry. I think my lasagna will fill your empty stomach."

Her home was filled with photos of family members. Remnants of a child's Lego creation sat in the corner. Removing my shoes despite Linda's protest, I shuffled to the kitchen where Lisa sat on a kitchen stool.

The conversation flowed like we had seen each other the day before. I felt myself relax and laugh, something I hadn't done in a while. However, I had to blink my eyes to stay awake. I knew I had to ask the next questions, but was embarrassed by it.

"Linda," I spoke above a whisper. "Is it okay if I lay on your couch?"

"Are you okay?" she immediately went into mother mode.

"I'm fine," not wanting to draw attention to myself. "But ever since surgery, I tire easily. I just need to rest a bit."

"Of course."

I slid down from the kitchen stool and sprawled on her comfortable couch. Within minutes, she handed me a blanket and a pillow.

"Go to sleep. Lisa and I will be right here, " she said pointing to the kitchen.

As a child, I used to love when my mother vacuumed and I was on the couch. Something about the repetitious sound lulled me to sleep. Friends' voices had the same effect. I don't know how long I slept, but the warmth of the blanket coupled with the scent of Italian food and the security of true friends helped me forget I was recovering from major surgery.

My Lesson Learned

After surgery, I know how important it is to make that phone call to let someone know you're thinking of him or her. I hope I don't forget that lesson.

May 25, 2019 - Check-up Echo

Does a broken heart mend? I feel scared. My fear is manifesting as a deep sadness. Life continues to happen while I wait for my next medical test. Picture a bottomless pit, I'm close to the base. My son left this morning for a 3-week stay in South Africa. That always puts me on edge. Today I go for my 2-year echocardiogram exam. I'm not afraid of the test. There's no pain associated with it. All I have to do is lay on my right side while a cold disc moves around my heart area. During the exam, I entertain myself by running movies with happy endings in my head.

When the operator turns up the volume, I know I'll hear the *swish, swish* sound of my valve opening and closing. I've learned not to ask what the sound means since I've heard the response before. "That's your valve opening and closing."

Today I get answers to a question I've kept buried. How is my heart doing? Did it get any worse?

Taking an ordinary walk is much more appreciated since I vividly recall being attached to medical machines and having to ask permission to urinate. I treasure inhaling the scent of roses. I can vividly recall inhaling the aroma of antiseptic. I wish my sense of taste would return. On the occasion my palate senses flavor, I'm thankful. In another 2 hours I'll know the condition of my heart.

***

The waiting room in this new office is large. Whatever germs are hiding remain invisible. There is plenty of room to spread out and I avoid any coughers.

"Joanna?" I hear my name called close to my 12:30 appointment.

Gathering my book, I stand up, "I'll be right there."

"My name is Cassie and I'll be doing your echo," she walked ahead of me. I feel like an obedient dog trailing behind awkwardly holding my book in my arm.

"Right here," she pointed to a room. "You can keep your shoes on. Undress from the waist up and tie the gown in the back," she said pointing to the garment.

Unfortunately, I know the routine. So I just smile and nod.

"I'll be back in a few minutes," she said as she gently shut the door.

Here we go again. I'm faced with uncertainty. I glance at the medical equipment that will be used to diagnose my heart's condition. I peek at the echo machine and see my name and date of birth in the left hand corner. It's flashing. I shiver. I should be use to it. I'm not.

Cassie returns and the test begins. A cold gel on a disc moved around my heart area. As her left hand maneuvers the disc, her right clicks on the computer mouse at different intervals. Since I'd know results within an hour, I try to remain calm. Getting hyper isn't going to do me or the results any good. Less than 20 minutes later, Cassie says, "That's it, get dressed. When you come out, I'll show you where to go to talk to Dr. Heart."

I hear a few more clicks on the echo machine and she leaves taking her bouncy brown curls with her.

As I dress, I peer at the monitor. There it is in the left hand corner. My name and date of birth. This time the information isn't flashing. All the test results are concealed in its mind's eye. Soon, it will be unlocked.

My mind, without my consent flashes back to my son's 12-hour flight to South Africa. When a worry subsidies, why does another concern automatically takes it place?

I open the door and Cassie leads me to another room. Here I sit trying to swat my apprehension away.

My Lesson Learned

I wish I knew why my mind goes to the worst case scenario. Am I programmed wrong?

Echo Result May 2019

I don't think I'll ever get used to staying in a room waiting for a doctor's results. No matter how inviting the room looks; I see danger lurking around the corner.

I sat on the examining table, my legs hanging down. It reminded me of a simpler time when as a child, my feet didn't touch the floor and life was easier.

Muffled sounds seeped through the bottom of the door. Noises that normally go unnoticed became louder than usual to my ears. The air-conditioning clicked on and then the sound of a fan.

A slight knock on the door, Dr. Heart came in and extended his hand.

"Nice to see you again, Joanna," he said.

"I wish I could say the same. But seeing you reminds me of my bad heart."

"Actually your heart is doing good. How are you feeling?"

"I feel fine, except for the fact I have no stamina."

"What do you mean?" he probed.

"Well, I'm a Pickleball player and I can't play two games in a row. I need to take a break."

He ran his fingers through his hair. "Why is that a problem?"

"I'm playing with people my age, but also people older than I. They don't rest. I get winded."

"Are you drinking anything?"

"Yes."

"What are you drinking?" he asked.

"I have lemonade with lots of water to keep the sugar content down."

"Have you thought of taking something with minerals and vitamins?" he questioned.

"Never thought of it. What would I drink?"

He gave me suggestions. I wrote them all down.

"Any other symptoms?" Dr. Heart asked.

"I feel when I try and take a deep breath, it's shallow, like I can't get enough air."

"Hmmm, when does that happen?"

"There's no rhyme or reason," I answered.

Without saying anything, I can tell he was considering options.

"Anything else?"

"Well, I don't want to sound like a hypochondriac, but I have another issue. My husband and I walk a lot. When I go up a hill, I have to stop, catch my breath for a few minutes and then continue."

"That sounds normal," he said. "Hills can do that."

"Yeah, but my husband is not out of breath, and he has 2 dogs yanking him."

"Okay. Would you be willing to take a stress test?"

"Yes," I replied.

"Set up an appointment and I'll go over the results with you the same day."

I hesitated, but only for a second.

"Can you make the appointment with me? They usually make me wait a couple of hours to see you for results."

He quickly said, "That's unnecessary. Let's go make the arrangements together."

With that, we talked to the receptionist and everything went seamlessly.

My Lesson Learned

Don't be afraid to ask for what you need. If I hadn't asked, I would have waited two hours for results.

June 6, 2019

"We're going to try to get your heart rate up to 130. Right now it's 82," said Jessica, the nurse who administered my stress test on the treadmill.

Before Jessica came in the room, Erica, another technician, asked me to undress from the waist up. Using alcohol she cleaned my chest area. Then she began to place sticky electrodes on me. She hooked the leads, but the confused expression on her face had me believe something was amiss. I was right.

"I'll be right back, just have a seat."

"Can you grab my book for me?" I pointed to my chair.

Within minutes Erica was back with another professional who did not give me her name.

"Let me take a look," as she glanced at the leads and began removing and rearranging them.

I reflected on being in a new position. I don't know that Erica was new, but her conduct mirrored someone who hadn't done this before. I kept my thoughts to myself to make her less uncomfortable.

The mystery person left the room once she was satisfied of the placements she made.

Jessica said, "I'm going to start you slow on the treadmill and every two minutes there will be an increase until your heart reaches 130 beats a minute. Are you ready?"

"Get 'er rolling," I said.

"Make sure you keep your feet at the top. Ready?" she asked

"Yes." I was very aware of keeping my feet at the top of the treadmill and never asked why I had to do that.

After two minutes, speed and incline increased. I handled it like a champ.

"I'm going to increase the speed and incline, are you okay?"

"Yes," I said a little winded. "But I can do it."

There was nothing to it. Sometimes I find myself making bigger issues out of matters that don't need space in my head. The only stress for the 'stress' test was self-imposed thinking beforehand.

"So, when will I see Dr. Heart ?" I asked as the speed began to decline.

"Oh, that won't be necessary. I can tell you. There is nothing abnormal about your test. In fact it's very good. But I will put these results on Dr. Heart's desk. If he sees anything, he will call you immediately."

Jessica rattled off my phone number. "Is that correct?"

"Yes," I answered.

"How soon does he see the results?" I inquired.

"Right after the patient he's with, so, about 15 minutes. Don't worry, everything looks good."

With that Erica removed all the leads with much more confidence than she put them on with. I got off the treadmill and continued on with my day. I don't think I'll ever get used to having heart-related tests.

My Lesson Learned

Someone said, 'Worry is like rocking in a chair and expecting to get somewhere. I need to get off the chair.'

March 31, 2020 – A Sense of Urgency

I had stabbing pains in my heart. My May appointment was just around the corner. Should I try to change it? At first, I did what I usually do, ignore it. But the pains had another intention. They kept coming. I mentioned the intensity to my husband who is not an alarmist. But he said, "Maybe you should call and see what Dr. Heart says." He paused a minute, "Have you taken the baby aspirin today?"

"No, I forgot." I tend to do that when I'm symptom free.

"Well, maybe you should. Take 2, it won't hurt you."

I found the orange-flavored chewable baby aspirin and nibbled on them.

Sitting in my back glass room I watched the birds freely come and go. They swooped down and ate the suet I left for them. Their chirping soothed me. I hoped the pain would subside by distracting myself. It didn't. I picked up the phone and called the cardiology office.

"Doctors Office, can you please hold? We're experiencing more calls than usual. If you'd like a call back, press the star key."

Sounds good to me. I pressed the star key.

The computer voice rattled off my phone number. "We'll call you back when you're next in queue. Please hang up."

No sooner had I hung up, the phone rang again.

"This is the cardiologist office. Your position is 2. Please hold."

I gathered a blanket my mother had crocheted before her death. It had holes in it now. I remember her spending hours putting it together. Her fingers grew tired, but her persistence wouldn't let her quit. I took this time to repair a few holes and felt warmth touching the yarn she had so lovingly held. I put my nose to the yarn to try and smell my mom's scent.

As I repaired each stitch, it reminded me of my repaired heart. Or was it repaired? *Had the stitching come undone like in the blanket I was repairing?*

"Your position is 1," the computer voice reminded me.

Join, stitch, join, stitch, I continued on and noticed the pain had not only subsided, it was gone. Should I just hang up? Something told me to stay on the line.

10 minutes later, I heard, "This is Ann, how may I help you?"

I really hope you can, I thought. My nerves were winning.

"Must be busy there today?" I questioned.

"I don't know, I just got here," she laughed. "How can I help you?"

I explained what happened.

"How long do these pains last?"

"It varies. Today was 10 minutes."

"What were you doing?"

"Nothing, just sitting reading a book."

"Has this happened before?"

"Yes, but I ignored it."

"How many times would you say during a week this has happened?"

"It's so intermittent. It could happen on Monday, then again on Wednesday and maybe twice on Wednesday. There's no rhyme or reason."

"Shortness of breath? Nauseousness?" she asked.

"No, just a sharp pain."

"Okay, I'm going to forward this information to Dr. Heart and I'll get back to you."

"In a day? In an hour?" I questioned.

"Oh, probably within the hour," she replied.

"Thank you," and with that we hung up.

I turned to the blanket and continued fixing the holes that happened due to wear and tear. I wonder if I have something in common with this blanket.

Within an hour, the phone rang and I was asked if I could come in today at two o'clock for some tests.

"I'll be there," I paused. "And thank you."

"You're welcome," she said.

I continued mending the blanket. I watched a woodpecker have a rhythm; a steady beat with his beak. I wanted the same tempo for my heart.

When I try to put things on the back burner, the issues tend to flame forward on their own. Before going to the appointment, I had lunch and tried to do normal things. Since I'm good at ignoring pain, I'm also adept at hiding fear from myself and others.

Arriving at the cardiologist's office, I felt relieved and nervous. In an hour, I'd know what was happening inside my body. My husband and I sat in the waiting room for only minutes before my name was called.

"Joanna?"

"Yes, can my husband come?"

"Sure. Come in please. My name is Sami and I'll be seeing you before Dr. Heart does."

I sat on the examining table and my vitals were taken. Elevated blood pressure was no surprise to me. She then began placing electrodes around my chest and limbs for an EKG reading.

"Please try and remain still so I can gather accurate information," Sami asked.

No problem. I wasn't going anywhere.

As efficiently as she placed the electrodes, she removed them. I didn't bother to ask about results since I knew I wouldn't get an answer.

"I'll give the results to Dr. Heart and he'll be with you in a few minutes," she said as she backed out of the door.

Paul read his book. I read the wall. 'Your Heart and Angina,' 'Your Heart's Mitral Valve.' I sat there wondering what could I be doing differently? I do some sort of exercise six out of seven days. My diet is mainly fruits and vegetables. But then there's genetics. Both of my parents had heart issues. Some things are out of my control.

A slight knock on the door brought me back to reality. Dr. Heart walked in and we exchanged pleasantries. "Your EKG came back normal. Tell me about your symptoms."

I rehashed everything I had told the nurse on the phone.

"Shortness of breath? " he asked.

"No."

"Does the pain radiate down your arm, neck or back?"

"No."

"The pain you are describing sounds more muscular. But let's do an echo and stress test just to be sure. Come with me please."

Paul and I followed him out of the room. We were now in another waiting area. I watched the medical technician wipe down all the equipment I'd be using. Smart move keeping the door open so I could observe the procedure.

Shortly after, I heard, "Joanna?"

"Yes," I answered.

"Come in please. My name is Mari and I'll be doing your echo," she said with a genuine smile. "You've done this before, right?"

"Yeah, unfortunately I'm a pro at it."

Pointing to the gown, she said "Please remove your shirt and bra and put on the blue gown and tie it in the back."

I should offer to draw a step by step procedure to put on the wall for the next patient.

"I'll be right back when you're ready," Mari said.

Mari knocked before entering and she began giving me the echo.

As I lay there, I took the opportunity to think about people in my life. My parents, both deceased, never complained when adversity struck. I thought about my own bout of cancer and how I just plowed through it at the age of 38. I recall being told I had the 'good' cancer. Really? There's 'good' cancer. I'm not afraid to die, but I'm also unwilling to hasten my exit.

"Ready for the stress test?" she asked.

"Sure," I said returning to the present.

As if on cue, a nurse appeared.

"My name is Lori, and I'll be conducting the stress test. I'll be with you the entire time." She smiled as she connected electrodes to various parts of my body. "My goal is to get you up to 130 beats per minute. I'll be increasing the speed and the incline. But before I do, I'll tell you."

I nodded.

"Are you ready?"

"Ready as I'll ever be," I replied.

Lori cheered me on as if I was running a marathon with fellow participants.

Grabbing on to the bar in front of me, I took these moments to reflect on my heart journey. Since I'm not able to compare my heart to others, I didn't know anything was amiss. I have Dr. Primary to thank for not having a life with oxygen. Had I known that not everyone's heart drummed loudly, I probably would have done something sooner. Who knew?

It's so important to have an annual physical especially when feeling fine.

The incline and speed increased. My deep breathing brought me back to reality. Gasping for air, she warned me, "I'm going to stop the treadmill now. Then you need to quickly lay down so Mari can finish up the echo."

I did as I was told. Mari asked, "Can you take a breath and hold it please?"

I was gulping for air and she wanted me to hold it? Not sure how I did it, but I was successful.

"You did great Joanna," both Mari and Lori chimed in together.

I lay on the table inhaling deeply.

Lori spoke, "We're going to step out. I'm give the results to Dr. Heart and when you're dressed, he'll talk with you."

I looked around the room. Seeing my clothes, I put them back on and glanced at my surroundings. I saw medical equipment that just analyzed my heart. I put the hospital gown back on the table and left the room to be greeted by my husband who was patiently waiting.

Before I could get my coat on, Dr. Heart appeared.

"Everything looks great, Joanna. I'm more confident that the pains you experienced were muscular. Your heart is good," Dr. Heart said.

I took a deep breath and slowly exhaled. I don't understand how or why the stabbing pain happened. I had to trust the results. So far, Dr. Heart has been 100% accurate.

"Make an appointment for another year and I'll check up on you again. Nice seeing you again Joanna."

"You too, Dr. Heart," I answered.

With that we shook hands and parted.

And so life continues. I try to discount twinges and aches. I'll never know what caused and continues to stab my heart periodically. But I do know I'll never regret going for a 'healthy' annual physical.

My Lesson Learned

Find balance and composure.

Choose courage over fear.

Live

Glossary

Here are definitions for some of the medical terms that may be obscure for some readers.

ICU   Intensive Care Unit

ID   Identification card, usually a photo ID card

INR   International Normalized Ratio, a measure of how long it takes for blood to clot.

IV   Intravenous, usually referring to therapy.

PA   Physician's Assistant

PICC   Peripherally Inserted Central Catheter, usually used for long-term IV antibiotics, nutrition, medications, or blood draw.

VNA   Visiting Nurse (Association)

About The Author

Joanna Montagna Torreano retired after 38 years of teaching. She taught grades 3 and 4 at a Buffalo Catholic School. She then taught remedial reading for students in grades K-5 for the Niagara Wheatfield Central Schools. She also worked part-time at Niagara University educating college students on how to teach reading.

Before retiring, her first book was published, '500 Questions and Answers for the New Teacher: A Survival Guide.'

For the past 25 years, Joanna has produced and hosted her own television program for Lockport Community Television. Her show, 'Studio One' covers a variety of local topics to promote the community.

After retiring, she spends time volunteering. She helps at a food pantry and tutors students.

An unexpected health issue inspired the book that you are now holding.

Book Club Discussion Topics

With the complexities of medical care for serious illnesses and their treatments, what is your approach to understanding what the doctors, nurses, and technicians are really telling you? I'm sharing my experiences in each chapter and *My Lesson Learned* following each chapter.

Do you keep your annual physical appointment? Why or why not?

Whom would you bring to an office visit? Why that particular person?

If you don't understand what medical personnel are telling you do you ask them to explain it to you again? Why or why not?

If you don't agree with medical personnel, would you say something?

What lessons have you learned after going through your medical procedure?

Written From The Heart guides you in answering these questions. And maybe raises other questions for you to manage your health.

Made in the USA
Middletown, DE
19 April 2022